"This book is a vital source of information for all speech and language therapists. It is a critical resource for newly-qualified therapists, as having an easy-to-read book which clearly outlines the process of assessment, diagnosis, and therapeutic intervention is invaluable and efficient. This book makes excellent links between clinical work and theory, with case studies to provide evidence."

Aimee Hilson, *Speech and Language Therapist, Sarah Buckley Therapies Ltd*

NAVIGATING SPEECH SOUND DISORDERS IN CHILDREN

Navigating Speech Sound Disorders in Children is an easy-to-read resource which gives an overview of the whole area of speech sound disorders (SSDs) in children, covering assessment, diagnosis, treatment, and management, underpinned by the latest research in the field.

The book focuses on key information, providing helpful therapy tips and evidence-based, practical advice drawing on clinical research and the author's extensive experience. Presented in 50 bite-sized chunks, therapists can find and refer to information quickly and easily. Additional guidance and links to further reading are signposted throughout so that the reader can explore topics in more detail, and a wealth of case examples is included to illustrate each point and demonstrate real-life application.

Written by a specialist in the field, this book provides strategies for students and qualified speech and language therapists (SALTs) working with children who present with many different types of SSD. It is valuable reading for both students and less experienced SALTs, as well as seasoned clinicians.

Kathryn Murrell is the author of *Working with Childhood Apraxia of Speech* and is a specialist SALT in independent practice, as well as a clinical supervisor in SSDs.

NAVIGATING SPEECH AND LANGUAGE THERAPY

Navigating the field of speech and language therapy can seem overwhelming to students and newly qualified therapists. This series is designed to provide concise, entry-level summaries of key areas in speech and language therapy, providing a basic insight into a specific area of therapy. Comprising practical advice and guidance from experts in the field, the books cover topics such as assessment, therapy, psychological approaches, and onward referral. This is a useful tool for anyone new to speech and language therapy or building confidence in the field.

Navigating Speech Sound Disorders in Children
50 Essential Strategies and Resources
Kathryn Murrell

Navigating Trans Voicing
50 Tips, Techniques and Fundamentals for Speech and Language Therapists
Matthew Mills and Natasha Stavropoulos

Navigating Voice Disorders
Around the Larynx in 50 Tips
Carolyn Andrews

Navigating AAC
50 Essential Strategies and Resources for Using Augmentative and Alternative Communication
Alison Battye

Navigating Telehealth for Speech and Language Therapists
The Remotely Possible in 50 Key Points
Rebekah Davies

Navigating Adult Stammering
100 Points for Speech and Language Therapists
Trudy Stewart

NAVIGATING SPEECH SOUND DISORDERS IN CHILDREN

50 ESSENTIAL STRATEGIES AND RESOURCES

Kathryn Murrell

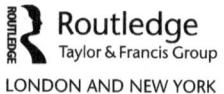

LONDON AND NEW YORK

Designed cover image: Getty Images

First published 2025
by Routledge
4 Park Square, Milton Park, Abingdon, Oxon OX14 4RN

and by Routledge
605 Third Avenue, New York, NY 10158

Routledge is an imprint of the Taylor & Francis Group, an informa business

© 2025 Kathryn Murrell

The right of Kathryn Murrell to be identified as author of this work has been asserted in accordance with sections 77 and 78 of the Copyright, Designs and Patents Act 1988.

All rights reserved. No part of this book may be reprinted or reproduced or utilised in any form or by any electronic, mechanical, or other means, now known or hereafter invented, including photocopying and recording, or in any information storage or retrieval system, without permission in writing from the publishers.

Trademark notice: Product or corporate names may be trademarks or registered trademarks, and are used only for identification and explanation without intent to infringe.

British Library Cataloguing-in-Publication Data
A catalogue record for this book is available from the British Library

ISBN: 9781032769851 (hbk)
ISBN: 9781032769837 (pbk)
ISBN: 9781003480778 (ebk)

DOI: 10.4324/9781003480778

Typeset in Aldus
by Deanta Global Publishing Services, Chennai, India

Dedication

In loving memory of Sarah Buckley (1976-2024) – beloved wife to Rob, inspirational speech and language therapist, gifted entrepreneur, chair of the Association of Speech and Language Therapists in Independent Practice, compassionate leader and manager, known and loved by friends and colleagues alike. You will continue to inspire all who knew you.

CONTENTS

List of Tables		xii
Acknowledgements		xiii
	Introduction	1

Part I
CLASSIFICATION AND SUBTYPES 3

1	What is a speech sound disorder?	5
2	How do we classify SSDs?	9
3	Phonological delay	13
4	Consistent phonological disorder	17
5	Inconsistent phonological disorder	19
6	Articulation disorder	21
7	Childhood apraxia of speech	27
8	When these subtypes overlap	33

Part II
ASSESSMENT AND DIAGNOSIS 37

9	Case history taking	39
10	The core speech sample	43
11	Detailed speech assessment	48
12	Transcription	52
13	Oral examination/oromotor screen	57
14	The pre-verbal child	62
15	Assessing the impact on the child's activity and participation	67
16	Assessing non-speech areas	72
17	The case profile and diagnostic statement	79
18	Communicating with others	86

Part III
TREATMENT 89

19	Goal-setting	91
20	Evidence-based practice	94
21	Choosing an intervention	99
22	The central role of parents/carers	104
23	Pre-verbal interventions	108
24	Phonological approaches: interventions with a strong evidence base	114
25	Phonological approaches: syllable-level intervention	121
26	Intervention for inconsistent phonological disorder	125
27	Therapy for articulation disorder: principles	132
28	Therapy for articulation disorder: common sound errors	138
29	Treatment approaches for CAS	143
30	Phonological awareness intervention	153
31	Working with older children with SSDs	156
32	Considerations for children from culturally and linguistically diverse backgrounds	159
33	Multiple areas of need	161
34	Outcome measures	166

Part IV
SERVICE DELIVERY AND DECISION-MAKING 169

35	Timing of therapy	171
36	Dosage	175
37	Discharge: when and how?	180
38	Effective time management	185
39	Caseload prioritisation	188
40	Group therapy	191
41	Blocks and breaks approach	193
42	Telehealth	196
43	Consultative approach	202

Part V
THE LINK WITH EDUCATION — **207**

44	Working in the school setting	209
45	EHCPs and report-writing	216
46	SEND tribunals	221
47	The link with literacy	227

Part VI
CONCLUDING THOUGHTS — **233**

48	The concept of 'disorder'	235
49	Where we are heading with SSDs	238
50	Moving forward with confidence	242

Index — **247**

TABLES

2.1	Cascade model of speech output processing	12
3.1	Common phonological processes and their approximate ages of elimination in typical acquisition (years, months)	15
6.1	Age of acquisition of English consonants	24
7.1	A comparison of CAS versus IPD	30
7.2	Characteristics of CAS versus childhood dysarthria	31
27.1	Summary of stages of articulation therapy principles	136

ACKNOWLEDGEMENTS

I would like to thank Jane Madeley and Molly Kavanagh from Taylor & Francis for enabling me to write this book.

I would also like to thank my husband, Ian, and our children – Hannah, Lucy, and Dom – for their unstinting support and encouragement.

INTRODUCTION

Navigating Speech Sound Disorders in Children is written for speech and language therapists (SALTs) and assistants, students, and other professionals who work with children with a speech sound disorder (SSD), such as teachers and special needs coordinators, as well as parents.

Unintelligible speech, or speech which is hard to understand, is often the first and most noticeable sign that a child has a communication impairment and is a very common reason for initial referral for a speech and language therapy assessment, accounting for 40% of all child referrals. Recently, there has been renewed interest in SSDs due to the development of many new treatments, and there is demand among SALTs for courses and supervision in SSDs – especially as this is a complex and controversial area, with different theoretical viewpoints suggesting different therapy approaches. The plethora of research into different types of SSDs over the last few years is transforming the way in which we view these disorders and promoting a greater understanding of the subgroups within the overall umbrella term 'speech sound disorder'. There have also been some changes in the terminology used in the UK, which are important to understand to ensure that we are clear, consistent, and accurate in our use of labelling and terms.

The complex nature of SSDs and their potential long-term effects on other aspects of development – such as literacy, educational attainment, and psychosocial development – highlight the importance of having skilled practitioners who are fully equipped to assess, diagnose, and treat children effectively.

This book aims to bring together all aspects of SSDs in a user-friendly resource which is based on the latest research but remains accessible and readable so that it can be dipped into without needing an advanced or specialist level of background knowledge. It provides SALTs and others with information on theoretical aspects, assessment and diagnosis, treatment, and clinical decision-making, and is in line with current recommendations from the Royal College of Speech and Language Therapists (RCSLT). The link between theory and practice is made throughout the book, and case studies are used as examples. As this is such a broad area of practice, it is not possible to provide extensive amounts of detail on every aspect of SSDs, so therapists are signposted to key texts, therapy resources, assessments, and websites for further information and training.

The book is divided into 50 short sections, allowing readers to dip in and out as necessary, and each section is complete in itself for quick and easy reference.

Readers are encouraged to become more confident, effective practitioners with children who have SSDs, as well as being inspired to explore further.

PART I

CLASSIFICATION AND SUBTYPES

Chapter 1

WHAT IS A SPEECH SOUND DISORDER?

WHICH CHILDREN ARE WE TALKING ABOUT?

Before launching into the area of SSDs, we need to know the population of children to which we are referring – and to be aware of those to whom this book does not refer.

Almost half of all children referred to SALTs have a primary difficulty with speech sounds, so it is vital that therapists are fully equipped – in terms of knowledge, understanding, and skills – to know how to approach this large cohort of children who come our way.

'Speech sound disorder' is an umbrella term, used internationally, that refers to children with any difficulty or combination of difficulties in perceiving, phonologically representing, and/or articulating speech, impacting speech intelligibility and acceptability, not typical of a child's age. It is also possible that the SSD may continue into adulthood, although children are the focus of this book. Although this may seem a little confusing, the term 'disorder' also includes children who have 'delayed' speech; this is discussed further in later sections in this part of the book. The RCSLT produced a guidance paper on SSDs in 2024 and agreed, through consultation with SALTs, that the term 'disorder' should be used in order to convey the seriousness and complexity of the condition. Use of the terms 'difficulty' and 'impairment' in the context of SSDs is not recommended, so throughout this book the term 'disorder' is used instead.

The focus of this book is primarily on children with SSDs where there is no known origin; however, specific populations of children are also mentioned, such as those with hearing loss or cleft palate. There are many children whose SSD has a known primary cause, which may be neurological, structural, or sensory, and some of these deserve a book in their own right. Some of these areas are considered 'specialities' and SALTs are advised to seek out further training before taking on some of these complex cases. One example is cleft palate, for which there are regional centres that usually have their own SALT team with the necessary high-tech equipment for assessment and therapy, as well as access to the whole cleft palate team. However, local therapists should be equipped to work with children who have a variety of complex aetiologies when there are more experienced, specialist SALTs available to provide the necessary support, either locally or from specialist teams. Hearing loss is another area of specialism and the RCSLT has information on its website for therapists interested in this area. However, many children with a history of fluctuating hearing loss due to glue ear may have phonological and/or articulatory difficulties with their speech, and these children can usually be treated using similar approaches to those used with children without a history of hearing problems.

The population of children with SSDs is very diverse in terms of:

- Aetiology (there may or may not be a known cause).
- Level of breakdown (e.g., input level, phonological representation, or articulatory level).
- Age of referral.
- The type of speech difficulties present.
- Severity.
- The need for the use of alternative and augmentative communication.
- The effect on intelligibility.
- The effect on communication, relationships, self-esteem, and overall functioning.
- The presence of additional, co-existing communication impairments.
- The presence of additional areas of need.

This book discusses children across the whole spectrum of ages, levels of severity, types of disorder, and the effect of the SSD on the child. For more complex, specialist areas, SALTs are signposted to further information and ways of accessing training in these fields. Diverse real-life case studies are also provided throughout, to illustrate many of the therapy techniques, approaches, and case management strategies.

WHO IS THIS BOOK FOR?

This book is intended to provide a broad overview of SSDs. It is thus primarily written for SALT students, those on apprenticeship schemes, newly qualified SALTs, SALT assistants, and therapists returning to practice, as well as more experienced therapists who want an overview of where we are as a profession in the field of SSDs or who wish to specialise in this area. This is a rapidly changing field and even in the last ten years there have been profound changes in the thinking on SSDs, how we classify children, the terminology used, and the evidence base for therapy techniques. This book is intended as a compact handbook which covers all aspects of SSDs, rather than a detailed exploration of research findings. Key texts are presented throughout so that therapists can find further information on specific issues. This book will also be useful for specialist teachers and other professionals who work with children with SSDs in mainstream schools and specialist provisions.

A plethora of books on the market address different aspects of SSDs – many from a comprehensive, academic perspective and others from a very practical perspective – to support parents and teachers in working with children with SSDs. This book, however, aims to provide practical guidance, based on up-to-date research and a strong evidence base. It is acknowledged that there are different opinions in the field of SSDs around classification, the theoretical framework, and approaches to therapy; however, this book is primarily written from a UK perspective and is rooted in current guidance from the RCSLT.

LAYOUT

There are 50 sections in this book, which are deliberately short to allow for easy digestion of the material and ensure that it can be dipped in and out of without losing the thread. Each section covers one area of SSDs and provides core information on that topic, with suggestions for practical application and references to key books or papers for further reading, as well as case studies where possible.

The sections are grouped into six parts, beginning with classification and subtypes, and moving onto assessment and diagnosis, treatment, service delivery and decision-making, the link with education, and concluding thoughts. The book ends with an invitation to explore further and to be bold in our approaches, not being afraid to try new things or to go outside our comfort zone.

USEFUL RESOURCES

The revised position paper on SSDs published by RCLST in 2024 is very comprehensive and can be found on its website at https://www.rcslt.org/news/new-speech-sound-disorders-guidance-published/

Chapter 2

HOW DO WE CLASSIFY SSDS?

Classification of SSDs has been a controversial and hotly disputed issue over the years, and as there is no universally agreed classification system, there has been considerable confusion over terminology – particularly regarding the use of the terms 'phonological disorder' versus 'articulation disorder'. The current preferred umbrella term to cover all types, irrespective of aetiology, is 'speech sound disorder', although sometimes the term 'speech impairment' is still used. For the purposes of this book, the preferred term in the UK – 'speech sound disorder' – is used throughout, as recommended by the RCSLT and as is also used internationally.

Falling within this umbrella term are several subgroups which we can identify using assessment techniques, although there are frequently overlaps between them and a child may not fit neatly into one subgroup.

The importance of identifying the subgroup(s) which best describe a child's speech patterns or features cannot be overemphasised, as this forms the basis of all clinical decisions about the type of intervention needed. It is also vital so that we can explain to parents and other professionals where the breakdown is happening and how we can address it.

CLASSIFICATION ACCORDING TO AETIOLOGY (OR 'CAUSE')

This uses the medical model to consider the cause or origin of the SSD. It is not a particularly useful way of looking at SSDs for therapists who are trying to identify the optimal intervention to use in treatment. Most children presenting with an SSD have no identifiable causal factor which accounts for the disorder, so this classification system is not helpful to us in these cases. Another term used for this is 'functional' – that is, of unknown cause.

Some children do have a known (or 'organic') cause for their SSD, including children with craniofacial differences (eg, cleft lip and/or palate or dental malocclusions), sensory impairments (eg, hearing loss), neurological disorder (eg, cerebral palsy), or Down's syndrome.

However, although it is important for us to know about these causal or possible causal factors, we are still left with questions about how to treat these children; and within what might look like a group with a single causal factor will be considerable variation, possible subgroups within these groups, and overlaps with other groups.

Just because a child might have a known 'cause', such as cleft palate, does not mean that all their speech difficulties can automatically be attributed to this. It may be that even if they did not have the cleft, they would still have an unrelated SSD. The causal model thus does not help us to get very far.

CLASSIFICATION ACCORDING TO LEVEL OF FUNCTIONING: THE BIOPSYCHOSOCIAL FRAMEWORK

This system was developed by the World Health Organization (WHO) to support the health and wellness of all people. It is a very useful tool for helping us to look at children with SSDs in terms of their body structure, body function, activities and participation, environmental factors, and personal factors. It can help us to see the child in their wider context and is very useful for setting goals and measuring outcomes.

PSYCHOLINGUISTIC CLASSIFICATION

Although several different classification systems have been attempted over the years, in this book we concentrate on the most common one, which was devised by Barbara Dodd. This classification is based on the speech output of real children, and the focus is on processing and output, rather than input (as this is often intact). This system identifies four distinct subtypes, plus childhood apraxia of speech (CAS), which are matched to areas of linguistic breakdown and are 'differentially diagnosable' – hence their popularity with SALTs. Children may, and frequently do, fit into more than one subtype and all children can be classified according to this method. Therapy can thus be targeted according to the subtype, based on the area of breakdown in the speech processing system. The RCSLT suggests that SALTs should use Dodd's labels and classification system – except what used to be called 'developmental verbal dyspraxia' should now be labelled 'childhood apraxia of speech', to reflect the change in UK terminology that was introduced in 2023.

Dodd devised the Diagnostic Evaluation of Articulation and Phonology (DEAP) assessment, which aims to identify the subgroup that best fits the child's speech characteristics so that therapy can be targeted accordingly. This assessment is very accessible and easy to carry out, and is recommended by the RCSLT as the 'gold standard assessment' for children with SSDs (according to the recently updated RCSLT SSD statement).

THE CASCADE MODEL

While many different models of speech processing have been proposed over the years, in this book we focus on the cascade model, which is a helpful way of looking at how speech sound processing works; we can then identify the possible area or areas of breakdown for a particular child. As we can see, there is not a simple one-to-one correspondence between the level of deficit and each of Dodd's subgroups, but this is explained in the following sections.

A more detailed explanation of how these levels of deficit affect the child's speech output – and thus our differential diagnosis – is given in Sections 3-8, where we cover each of Dodd's subgroups in turn.

SUBGROUPS WHICH CAN BE IDENTIFIED USING THE DEAP

- Phonological delay.
- Consistent phonological disorder (CPD).
- Inconsistent phonological disorder (IPD).

Table 2.1 Cascade model of speech output processing

	Level of deficit	Differential diagnosis
1	Phonological rules (error patterns are delayed or atypical)	Phonological delay/consistent phonological disorder
2	Phonological plan/template	Inconsistent phonological disorder
3	Phonetic programme assembly	Articulation disorder (Type I: substitution) (ie, with phonological consequences)
4	Motor speech programme implementation	Articulation disorder (Type II: distortion) or oral dyspraxia (motor speech programme disorder)
5	Execution of motor program	Dysarthria + anatomical problems (eg, clefts)
6	Multi-level deficits: phonological plan, phonetic programme assembly, and motor speech programme implementation	CAS

Source: Based on Ozanne, 2005.

- Articulation disorder.
- CAS.

The next five sections describe each of these in turn.

REFERENCES

Ozanne, A (2005). The search for developmental verbal dyspraxia. In: Dodd, B (ed). *Differential Diagnosis and Treatment of Children with Speech Disorder*. Whurr Publishers.

RCSLT (2024). New Speech Sound Disorder Guidance published. https://www.rcslt.org/news/new-speech-sound-disorders-guidance-published/

WHO (World Health Organization) (WHO Workgroup for development of version of ICF for Children) (2007) International Classification of Functioning, Disability and Health – Version for Children and Youth 2013-CY. Geneva" World Health Organization.

Chapter 3

PHONOLOGICAL DELAY

WHAT IS THE UNDERLYING DEFICIT?

Children with phonological delay have a delay or immaturity with their understanding of *phonological rules*. The correct rules are developing, but at a slower rate than would be expected. There is often no known cause for phonological delay, although there may be co-occurring factors such as hearing loss or developmental delay.

HOW DOES IT AFFECT SPEECH?

This group of children accounts for just over half of a typical SSD caseload. The child's speech sound system follows phonological rules (patterns) which are characteristic of a chronologically younger child, but has no unusual substitutions or error patterns that are not seen in typical speech development. Children may have just one delayed process or a small number operating simultaneously, and the effect on intelligibility will vary accordingly. Children with large amounts of phoneme collapse or older children with persistent delayed patterns may be classified as having CPD (note that this is a change in definition from the original Dodd diagnostic groups).

The result of phonological delay is the loss of *contrast* between sounds and thus between words. This means that a child with a combination of several delayed phonological processes might say, for example, [dɔ] to mean 'door', 'saw', 'core', and 'four'.

As the speech of children with phonological delay follows rules (patterns), we can usually predict how a child will produce a given word. This means that it is easier for a listener to 'tune in' to the child and interpret what they mean – especially if there are only one or two phonological processes operating and there are no other speech sound difficulties present.

The distinction between 'delay' and 'disorder' is important and we need to be familiar with typical speech acquisition – particularly the ages at which different phonological processes are evident – so that we can make decisions about whether a child's patterns are age appropriate, delayed, or disordered.

A QUICK RECAP OF COMMON PHONOLOGICAL PROCESSES

SOME IMPORTANT POINTS TO REMEMBER

- Children develop speech patterns gradually, so the ages of elimination of phonological processes should be seen as very approximate. When a child is moving towards using a more *mature* contrast, they will usually start using it *sometimes* and then gradually use it more *consistently* over time. There may thus be a time when they may, for example, be stopping [s] some of the time but using [s] appropriately at other times. The word 'sea' may therefore be produced as [ti] and [si] within the same conversation. Other factors which may affect how consistently the child uses the target sound include contextual factors (eg, length of word or utterance, speed of utterance) and other factors, such as whether the child is tired or thinking hard about their sound production. We need to be careful not to confuse this with *inconsistency*, which may lead us to think that the child has a disorder.
- There has been a recent consensus change to the original Dodd classification for phonological delay, which now states that children who have delayed phonology as they get older – and even into adulthood – are referred to as having 'phonological disorder'. This replaces the original definition, which was purely based on the nature of the child's output, without regard to their age.

Table 3.1 Common phonological processes and their approximate ages of elimination in typical acquisition (years, months)

Process	Description	Age
Context-sensitive voicing	A voiceless sound is replaced by a voiced sound eg, 'peg' /peg/ → [beg]	3;0
Word-final devoicing	A final voiced consonant is replaced by a voiceless one eg, 'beg' /beg/ → [bek]	3;0
Final consonant deletion	The final consonant in a word is omitted eg, 'boot' /but/ → [bu]	3;3
Velar fronting	A velar stop is replaced by an alveolar stop or nasal eg, 'cap' /kæp/ → [tæp]	3;6
Palatal fronting	The palato-alveolar fricatives /ʃ/ and /ʒ/ are replaced by alveolar fricatives /s/ and /z/ eg, 'shoe' /ʃu/ → /su/	3;9
Consonant harmony	Pronunciation of the whole word is influenced by the presence of a particular sound in the word e.g, 'bag' /bæg/ → [gæg]	4;0
Weak syllable deletion	Syllables are either stressed or unstressed e.g, 'because' /bəˈkɒz/ → [kɒz]	4;0
Cluster reduction	Part of the consonant cluster in a word is omitted e.g, 'blue' /blu/ → [bu]	4;0
Gliding of liquids	The liquid consonants /l/ and /r/ are replaced by the glides /w/ or /j/ e.g, 'leg' /leg/ → [jeg]	5;0
Stopping	A fricative or affricate consonant is replaced by a stop /f/, /s/ eg, 'soup' /sup/ → [tup] /v/, /z/ eg, 'zoo' /zu/ → [du] /θ/, /ð/ eg, 'theme' /θim/ → [tim]	3;0 3;6 5;0

Source: Grunwell, 1987.

- There may be a combination of delayed and disordered phonological processes at the same time; this is very common, if not the norm, in children with disordered phonology. In this case, we would categorise them as having a 'disorder' (either CPD or IPD) rather than a 'delay' as well. If a child with a disorder makes progress and is left with some residual 'delayed' processes, we can then classify them as having a 'delay'.
- To meet the criteria for 'phonological delay', a child should be able to produce all age-appropriate single sounds in isolation. If not, they have an additional *articulation disorder*. If a child is unable to produce a particular age-appropriate sound in isolation – for example, if they substitute [k] with [t] in all word positions – we would have to say at this stage that the main issue is with *articulation*, as we cannot yet tell whether there is also a *phonological* component. We can change the differential diagnosis to 'phonological delay' at a later stage if the child starts producing the target sound in isolation and in up to one position in a syllable (eg, [ɑk] or [kɑ]), but still substitutes [t] in place of [k] in other positions.

REFERENCES

Grunwell, P (1987). *Clinical Phonology* (2nd ed). Croom Helm.

Chapter 4

CONSISTENT PHONOLOGICAL DISORDER

WHAT IS THE UNDERLYING DEFICIT?

Children with CPD account for about 20% of SSD referrals. The level of deficit with this group of children is with phonological rules, as with phonological delay; but in this case, the child's phonological error patterns are atypical (non-developmental) – that is, they are not seen in the speech of typically developing children. Children have an impaired understanding of the phonological system.

Also included in this subtype (as a recent change to the original Dodd classification definition) are children with large amounts of phoneme collapse and older children with persistent delayed patterns.

HOW DOES IT AFFECT SPEECH?

As with phonological delay, the error patterns are consistent and predictable, which means that the child is sometimes reasonably intelligible, unless several processes are operating simultaneously. If the child is using multiple processes, even if they are consistent, the resulting speech may be highly unintelligible – particularly as their phonemic inventory is likely to be limited, which will cause loss of contrast. Also, if the *phonotactic* structure of the word is affected (ie, the permissible syllable structure, consonant clusters, and vowel sequences) – for example, deletion of all initial consonants – the child will be highly unintelligible, as every word will begin with a vowel. Children with CPD usually also have some delayed typical phonological processes in operation, but we do not use the term 'phonological delay' in addition to CPD for children who have both. Examples of atypical rules include gliding fricatives and initial consonant deletion.

Children with CPD can produce all age-appropriate sounds in isolation; if not, we would describe them as having an *articulation disorder* as well.

Case example

James was referred with unintelligible speech at age three and a half. His receptive and expressive language were age appropriate and no significant factors were raised in his case history. His hearing, when tested, was found to be normal. When assessed, it was found that he deleted all syllable-initial consonants except for 'm', which was used word-initially; however, he used consonants in VC position. His vowels were all appropriate. James also had word-final devoicing – for example, 'bag' was produced as 'ack'. This is a delayed phonological process. At the time of initial assessment, it was unclear whether James also had other delayed phonological processes, as he used such a limited range of initial consonants. As James used unusual speech sound substitutions consistently and had no signs of CAS or dysarthria, his SSD was diagnosed as CPD.

Chapter 5

INCONSISTENT PHONOLOGICAL DISORDER

WHAT IS THE UNDERLYING DEFICIT?

About 10% of children referred with SSDs have IPD. This is due to a deficit in the phonological plan, or template, which results in a combination of error types with variability of production of single words that is equal to or greater than 40%. Children with IPD have a deficit in the creation and storage of phonological representations.

HOW DOES IT AFFECT SPEECH?

Children with IPD have a combination of delayed and non-developmental speech errors, but it is the *inconsistency* of their errors, at word level, which distinguishes IPD from CPD. Repeated productions of the same word will be inconsistent in terms of consonants and vowels used, as well as phonotactic structures. It is important to measure the percentage of *inconsistency* of single word production; for a differential diagnosis of IPD, this is 40% or more. (This reflects the fact that there is often some degree of inconsistency anyway in children who do not have IPD.) Words may bear no resemblance to the target word, which causes speech to be unintelligible – even to close family members at times. There are usually also typical phonological processes as well as some consistent unusual phonological processes alongside the inconsistent ones.

Imitation is usually better than spontaneous production of a word, as the child is given the phonological representation, so they do not have to create it for themselves or store it. If they still produce errors on imitation (eg, with single sounds or words), either there may be other additional areas of speech disorder alongside IPD (eg, articulation disorder) or the differential diagnosis is incorrect. There is no obvious oromotor dysfunction with IPD.

Children with IPD often have highly unintelligible speech, but prosody and voice are unlikely to be affected. Their speech can be very complex to analyse, but an accurate differential diagnosis is essential because most types of therapy used to address other subtypes of SSDs are likely to be ineffective or to have very little impact. There is a strong evidence base in favour of using *Core Vocabulary Intervention* to treat this group of children (see Section 25).

CASE EXAMPLE

Noah was referred age two and a half due to very poor intelligibility and frustration felt by both child and parents that he could not get his message across, as well as expressive language delay, as he was not yet joining two words together. Assessment showed that he had approximately 50 single words; however, it was hard to know which word he was using, as there was a high level of inconsistency. His errors could not be analysed according to a series of predictable patterns and he often used sounds which were unrelated to the target sounds. Noah's difficulties with getting his message across resulted in frequent tantrums. Differential diagnosis was difficult at first and it was unclear whether he had either IPD or CAS; however, a tentative diagnosis of IPD was made and some therapy using CVI was used, which was very successful within several weeks. This confirmed the initial diagnosis of IPD and Noah became much more intelligible, although he had continued expressive language delay which needed ongoing therapy for the next year.

Chapter 6

ARTICULATION DISORDER

This is the inability to produce a perceptually acceptable version of a particular phoneme, either in isolation or in any phonetic context. 'Perceptually acceptable' is an important aspect, because we are focusing not on the accuracy of *how* a phoneme made but on how it *sounds* auditorily. For example, the phoneme /s/ may be produced with the tongue in a variety of positions for it to sound acceptable auditorily (eg, behind the upper or lower incisors).

There are two types of articulation disorder, which have different underlying deficits, as follows.

STRUCTURAL

This is when a structural deficit in the oro-dento-facial region results in sound distortion. Examples include cleft lip and/or palate malformations, velocardiofacial syndrome, and other cranio-facial syndromes. Cleft lip and/or palate is the most common congenital abnormality in the cranio-facial region and children usually have SSDs due to the cleft, which are often exacerbated by associated dental anomalies and an increased risk of hearing loss.

The underlying deficit is in the execution of the motor program. Articulation disorder caused by structural deficits is mentioned in this book in the assessment sections, in relation to differential diagnosis and when to refer for further investigations, but is not covered in detail as these are specialist areas.

FUNCTIONAL

This is most common form of articulation disorder. There is no known cause and oro-facial structures are intact.

There are two different presentations of functional articulation disorder, as follows.

TYPE I: SUBSTITUTION

In this case, the level of deficit is in the *phonetic programme assembly*. The deficit is *articulatory* in origin, but the child substitutes some sound for another which crosses the phonemic boundary and is thus perceived by the listener as a different sound. It is therefore an *articulatory deficit*, but with *phonological consequences*. This results in a meaningful contrast. It is crucial that the correct distinction is made between an SSD which is *articulatory* in origin as opposed to *phonological* in origin, as therapy for a Type I substitution disorder should be *articulatory* in nature because the child is unable to produce the target sounds in isolation or in segments.

EXAMPLE

If the child says 'cat' /kæt/ as [tæt] but is unable to imitate /k/ in isolation, this is an *articulatory* error with *phonological consequences*. If the child *can* produce /k/ in isolation and in *one but no more than one* of the following vocalic positions – CV, VC or VCV (eg, /kɑ/, /ɑk/ or /ɑkɑ/) – we can say that the deficit is *articulatory*.

TYPE II: DISTORTION

In this case, the level of deficit is at the level of *motor speech program implementation*. There is a variation in the child's realisation of the sound, but the listener still perceives it auditorily as the target sound. The sound is thus distorted due to inaccurate placement of the articulators, and the resultant sound is usually not an English sound or one used in another of the child's languages.

A breakdown at this *motor speech program implementation* level is also responsible for oral dyspraxia.

Children with distortion errors are usually intelligible, as there is no loss of contrast and the listener can usually tune in, but their speech may sound 'different' or 'unusual'.

Common distortion errors include:

- Dentalised, lateral, palatal, or nasal lingual fricatives (eg, /s/, /z/, /ʃ/).
- Distortions of /ɹ/, /θ/ and /ð/.

Some so-called 'errors' may be dialectal and we should be careful about labelling these as a 'disorder'. Issues around the concept of 'disorder' are discussed in Section 48. For example, in parts of the UK, the phoneme /θ/ is often realised as /f/; but rather than this being a substitution disorder, this may well be dialectal and may be appropriate for that child in their environment.

Interestingly, phoneticians are predicting that in 50-100 years, certain sounds may no longer be key in our inventory, as they are gradually being used less in the adult population and other sounds are being accepted in their place. Examples include the use of /f/ and /v/ in place of /θ/ and /ð/ and /ʊ/ in place of /r/.

A QUICK RECAP OF SPEECH SOUND ACQUISITION

These norms are approximate, rather than static over time, and are also subject to dialectal variation, so they are not recommended for use as the sole measure of whether a child's speech is age appropriate. As for the development of phonological processes (see Section 3), the acquisition of these consonants is gradual; therefore, while a child is slowly moving towards using one specific sound, there may be a period of inconsistency before they have generalised it fully into their spontaneous connected speech.

Table 6.1 Age of acquisition of English consonants

	50%	90%
/p/	18 months	3 years
/m/	18 months	3 years
/h/	18 months	3 years
/n/	18 months	3 ¼ years
/w/	18 months	3 years
/b/	18 months	3 years
/k/	2 years	3 ½ years
/g/	2 years	3 ¾ years
/d/	2 years	3 ¼ years
/t/	2 years	3 ¾ years
/ŋ/	2 years	7 years
/f-/	2 ½ years	3 ½ years
/-f/	2 ½ years	5 ½ years
/j/	2 ½ years	4 ½ years
/ɹ/	3 years	8 years
/l-/	3 years	5 ½ years
/-l/	3 years	6 ½ years
/s/	3 years	7 years
/tʃ/	3 ½ years	6 ½ years
/ʃ/	3 ½ years	6 ½ years
/z/	3 ½ years	7 years
/j/	4 years	6 ½ years
/v/	4 years	5 ½ years
/θ/	4 ½ years	7 years
/ð/	4 years	7 years
/ʒ/	5 years	8 years

Source: Combined data from a variety of sources, including Grunwell, 1981.

WHERE DOES DYSARTHRIA FIT IN?

Dysarthria is a neuromuscular motor speech disorder in which the muscles used to produce speech are damaged, paralysed, or weakened. The child finds it difficult to control and coordinate the speed, range, strength, and duration of movements needed for speech. This can make it harder to produce specific sounds and speech may be slurred or hard to understand. Childhood dysarthria is associated either with congenital disorders, such as cerebral palsy or syndromes (developmental), or with acquired aetiologies such as head injury, brain tumours, or strokes.

Dysarthria is due to a deficit at the level of *execution of motor program,* which is at the same level of breakdown as anatomical problems such as clefts.

Common characteristics of childhood dysarthria include:

- Poor control of respiration and/or shallow breathing.
- Poor quality of vocal fold vibration.
- Poor voice quality and prosodic difficulties, particularly affecting pitch and volume.
- Problems with resonance; often, excessive nasality.
- Poor control over lips and tongue, causing articulation difficulties.
- Consistent speech errors.
- Speech sound distortions due to weak articulatory contacts.

CASE EXAMPLE

Janey had a stroke in utero which caused mild cerebral palsy, expressive language delay, and unclear speech, as well as other health problems, including epilepsy. As there were several significant health concerns, apart from her speech, there was a delay in when she was referred for a SALT assessment. She was first seen at three years of age, when she had a few unclear single words. Assessment showed that Janey had age-appropriate receptive language and as she had a strong desire to communicate, she responded very well to signing initially. As her expressive language developed, the SALT sessions became more focused on speech production. She presented with consistent speech sound errors, with particularly noticeable slurring and weak articulatory contacts, and she was mildly hypernasal. Janey's overall speech was slow and effortful, and she struggled to produce accurate sounds in isolation, in words, and in conversation. DEAP assessment showed that there was no phonological element to her speech and perceptually, she had many features of developmental dysarthria, which could be attributed to her stroke in utero. No obvious phonological features were found to be present.

REFERENCES

Grunwell, P (1981). The development of phonology. *First Language*, iii, 161–191.

Chapter 7

CHILDHOOD APRAXIA OF SPEECH

WHAT IS THE UNDERLYING DEFICIT?

CAS (formally known as 'developmental verbal dyspraxia' in the UK until 2023) is the least common type of SSD, found in under 1% of children with SSDs. CAS is classified as a 'multi-level' deficit disorder, as the breakdown is thought to be at three levels: the phonological plan, phonetic programme assembly, and motor speech programme implementation.

There is general agreement that the nature of the impairment is neurological, without damage to muscles or nerves. The American Speech and Hearing Association (ASHA) provides the following definition:

> Childhood apraxia of speech is a childhood neurological speech disorder in which the precision and consistency of movements underlying speech are impaired in the absence of neuromuscular deficits. The core impairment in planning and/or programming the spatio-temporal parameters of movement sequences results in errors in speech sound production and prosody.

WHAT ARE THE SPEECH CHARACTERISTICS?

CAS is the most complex and controversial subgroup in the field of SSDs and there have been many years of discussion, debate, and disagreement about the nature of this disorder, how to diagnose it, and how to distinguish it from other SSDs which share similar characteristics.

ASHA and the RCSLT have both published excellent position papers on CAS and there are three consensus characteristics agreed by both as the minimum necessary for a diagnosis of CAS. However, as yet there is no validated set of diagnostic criteria on which to base a diagnosis of CAS, as these characteristics can also be found in other SSDs. Diagnosis depends on expert judgement of perceptual features, so a skilled and experienced therapist is needed for accurate diagnosis.

The consensus characteristics are as follows:

- Inconsistent errors on consonants and vowels in repeated productions of syllables or words.
- Lengthened or disrupted co-articulatory transitions between sounds and syllables or words.
- Inappropriate prosody, especially in the realisation of lexical or phrasal stress.

The child must also have a clear intent to communicate.

A note of caution should be given at this point regarding the three consensus characteristics, as the degree to which these are present or observed is also affected by the age of the child and the extent of their verbal output. This applies in particular to inconsistency, which may not be obvious in a child who has limited verbal output.

There are also many other features which are frequently reported in the speech of children with CAS, including slow diadochokinetic rate (DDK), vowel distortion, increased errors with longer words and utterances, articulatory 'groping' during sound production, late or absent babble, and imitation worse than spontaneous speech. The feature of 'groping', which is often documented, is more likely to be obvious in a child with severe CAS who is attempting to imitate, rather than in spontaneous speech.

As diagnosis is not always easy or clearcut, it is sometimes suggested that, rather than labelling a child with CAS prematurely, we use the term 'suspected CAS' if we are unsure. In such cases, it is important that therapy is initiated as soon as possible, rather than waiting for a firm diagnosis; and the child's response to the therapy we choose will also inform our diagnosis.

Although CAS is a rare disorder and is thus a 'low-incidence' condition, it is also considered a 'high-need' condition, as children with CAS usually need the highest level of SALT input out of all the groups of children we see with SSDs.

PROBLEMS WITH OVER-DIAGNOSIS

CAS is notoriously over-diagnosed – mainly because the characteristics overlap with other SSDs – and it may also co-exist with other types of disorders. The problem with misdiagnosis is that the therapy approach chosen will be incorrect and is unlikely to be effective. CAS requires a very different type of approach from IPD, although these are often confused.

DIFFERENTIATING CAS FROM IPD

Table 7.1 A comparison of CAS versus IPD

CAS	IPD
Level of breakdown Multi-level deficits at the level of motor programming and planning. The breakdown is at the output side of the speech processing model.	*Level of breakdown* The creation and storage of phonological representations.
Speech features Inconsistent production of consonants, vowels, and phonotactic structures on repeated productions of the same word.	*Speech features* Inconsistent production of consonants, vowels, and phonotactic structures on repeated productions of the same word. Difficulties in maintaining consistent production in spontaneous speech, being inconsistent in at least half the words produced. Many atypical errors, with few systemic error patterns being apparent.
Consonant and vowel errors on imitation	No difficulty in imitating age-appropriate vowels and consonants.
Limited phonotactic structures.	No challenges with repeating age-appropriate phonotactic structures and words, unless the child has co-occurring articulatory difficulties.
Lengthened and disrupted co-articulatory transitions between sounds and syllables; inappropriate prosody, particularly stress; and noticeable gaps between syllables.	Prosody unlikely to be affected.
Overall lack of clarity and precision.	
Increased difficulty with production of polysyllabic words.	
Fluency and/or voice may be affected.	Fluency and/or voice unaffected unless there is a co-occurring difficulty.
Imitation is poorer than spontaneous production.	Imitated speech is closer to the target production than spontaneous speech.
Phonological awareness Usually unaffected.	*Phonological awareness* Likely to have an associated deficit in phonological awareness.

(Continued)

Table 7.1 Continued

CAS	IPD
Oromotor or feeding difficulties Children may well have difficulties in this area.	*Oromotor or feeding difficulties* Rarely present.
DDK Slow DDK rate and sequencing (eg, producing 'p-t-k' in quick succession).	*DDK* Within the normal range.

Source: Combined data from RCSLT, 2024 and ASHA, 2007.

DIFFERENTIATING CAS FROM CHILDHOOD DYSARTHRIA

These two types of speech disorder are very hard to tell apart and may also co-exist. Table 7.2 highlights some of the characteristic differences to look out for. As the presence or absence of these characteristics relies on the perceptual observations of the therapist, it requires a certain level of skill and experience to make an accurate diagnosis.

Table 7.2 Characteristics of CAS versus childhood dysarthria

Speech features	CAS	Childhood dysarthria
Weakness	No weakness, incoordination, or paralysis of speech musculature.	Reduced strength and/or coordination of speech musculature.
Inconsistency of speech errors	Inconsistent errors.	Consistent errors.
Types of speech sound error	Speech sound substitutions, omissions, and additions.	Speech sound distortions due to weak articulatory contacts.
Resonance	May have inconsistent resonance due to mistiming.	Hypernasal resonance common.
Voice quality	May have breathy or hoarse voice.	Poor control of pitch and volume. May have an atypical voice quality.
Prosody	Prosodic difficulties affecting stress, rhythm, and rate.	Prosodic difficulties affecting rhythm and rate.

Source: ASHA, 2007.

CASE EXAMPLE

Aaron was referred at four years of age with moderately delayed expressive language and unintelligible speech. His receptive language was age appropriate. Aaron had obvious signs of difficulties with motor coordination and frequently fell off his chair during the initial assessment. He used lots of self-taught gestures to communicate and managed to communicate with familiar adults using these gestures, although he needed his mother to interpret when he spoke to unfamiliar adults. Assessment showed severe difficulties with imitating sounds and words, and with imitating oral movements. His connected speech was slow and he used equal stress for each syllable, as well as adding a schwa at the ends of many words. Aaron also had some social communication differences; however, the focus of therapy was on developing his intelligibility. His period of assessment coincided with the Covid-19 pandemic, so sessions had to move online, which meant that a differential diagnosis was more difficult. However, he was given a diagnosis of CAS and subsequently an autism spectrum disorder (ASD) diagnosis.

REFERENCES

ASHA (2007). Childhood apraxia of speech (technical report). www.asha.org/policy/tr2007-00278/

RCSLT (2024). Position paper on childhood apraxia of speech (CAS). www.rcslt.org/wp-content/uploads/2024/02/RCSLT-Childhood-Apraxia-of-Speech-CAS-Position-Paper-2024.pdf

Chapter 8

WHEN THESE SUBTYPES OVERLAP

Things would be much more straightforward if every child fitted neatly into one diagnostic 'box'. The Dodd classification should not be seen in this way, however, as there is a universal recognition that children often have a mixed profile which involves aspects of two or more subtypes. It may also be the case that a broad diagnostic label can cover *different* underlying impairments and in this case, there may be an 'umbrella' within each diagnostic category.

In practice, many children referred due to concerns over their speech sound production appear to have difficulties with both articulation and phonology. Other children who may have obvious features of CAS can also have features of dysarthria. It can sometimes seem overwhelmingly complex to work out exactly what is going on with a particular child. One way of trying to work this through is by identifying the primary subtype and focusing on treating that first; or they can be worked on simultaneously. We should identify which aspect of a child's SSD is having the most severe effect on their communication, which may also be the one that has the greatest impact on their intelligibility. If a child has a substitution articulation disorder and is struggling to produce certain key sounds, it is important to work on this first, before we can determine whether there is also a phonological component to the disorder.

In this situation, we should use a flexible approach and gather information over time to help us to see the full picture. We can always revise our initial diagnosis later, as the way in which a child responds to therapy always informs the ongoing diagnostic process. Our messaging to parents, carers, schools, and other professionals is crucial. We should state the things we know, using a diagnostic label if possible, but make it clear that as time moves on and therapy progresses, our understanding may change. For example, a young child may have obvious CAS features in the early stages, but as therapy progresses, a CAS diagnosis may no longer be appropriate. We can thus revise the initial diagnosis in line with their progress in therapy, as the presenting characteristics of the SSD evolve.

Certain subtypes are often commonly associated and co-occur more than others. For example, phonological delay and articulation disorder often go together, as do CAS and childhood dysarthria. Phonological delay is often a feature of all the other subtypes, but we would not include this as part of the diagnostic label.

It is also helpful for us to be aware that speech development is *dynamic* – that is, areas interact over time and there is a combination of both motor and linguistic factors. For example, a child with phonological delay who fronts their velars in all word positions will not have the opportunity to practise producing velar sounds, which may have consequences for their *motor* speech development. There may also be a *phonological* consequence of a *motor* problem.

Case examples

Phonological delay + articulation disorder (substitution)

Jo presented at four years of age with fronting of all velars and stopping of 'f' to 'b' in all word positions. He was able to produce velar sounds in isolation and could imitate them accurately in CV and VC positions (providing evidence that this was a phonological substitution). However, he struggled to produce an accurate 'f' in isolation and used 'b' in place of 'f' (articulatory substitution error). He received some direct one-to-one therapy using alveolar/velar minimal pairs, and after eight sessions he was consistent with the velar/alveolar contrast in single words. He found it very difficult to learn accurate production of 'f', which took several weeks; however, he managed to achieve it and as soon as he could produce 'f' in isolation, he was confident enough to continue working through the hierarchy of increasing levels of difficulty until he achieved 'f' in conversation.

CAS + dysarthria

Will had a stroke in utero and presented with a left hemiplegia, a history of feeding difficulties, and a complex speech profile which included a high level of vowel and consonant inconsistency, poor overall intelligibility, prosodic difficulties, slowed rate, and a consistently slurred speech quality, with some consistent hypernasality. Differential diagnosis was difficult; but due to his consistent hypernasality and slurred speech, alongside inconsistency with vowel and consonant production, which was more apparent in polysyllabic words, he received a working diagnosis of CAS and dysarthria.

Consistent phonological disorder + articulation disorder (distortion)

Aarav was referred at three years of age with some unusual substitutions ('sh' in place of 'g' and 'g' in place of 'd'). These substitutions were consistent but did not follow the usual developmental sequence. He also struggled to produce 'l' accurately and for this sound, his tongue protruded almost as far out as his upper lip. He could place his tongue in the correct place when shown, but he was unable to produce an accurate 'l' sound. His speech was, however, relatively intelligible, as he was consistent in connected speech. He was diagnosed with CPD and articulation disorder.

PART II

ASSESSMENT AND DIAGNOSIS

Chapter 9

CASE HISTORY TAKING

WHY IS THIS NEEDED?

- Case history-taking gives us essential background information about the child and their family. We can find out about the child's hearing status and their development in different areas.
- It can help with differential diagnosis, as we can ask questions about the child's early speech and language development, feeding and so on. Questions related to early indicators of a possible disorder such as CAS can be raised.
- Specific areas raised in the case history will affect the areas of assessment carried out – for example, whether a detailed oromotor assessment is needed.
- Any additional areas of concern can be raised which may need to be referred to another agency (eg, possible hearing problems).
- We can find out how the parent feels about their child's speech and ask about what strategies they use at home.
- We can ask how the child communicates in different environments and with different people (eg, home versus nursery, adults versus siblings).

HOW DO WE CARRY IT OUT?

The case history is an essential component of the assessment process and there are different ways in which it can be carried out, depending on the age of the child and the context of the assessment (eg, an older child with a mild speech sound difficulty versus an unintelligible four-year-old who appears to have a complex profile). Ideally, case history-taking should be in person with the parent/parents or carers, but sometimes this may not be possible or practical – especially if the child is being seen in school. Case histories may also be taken online, by phone, through questionnaires, or by email. If it is not possible to have access to the parents, schools may be able to provide essential information on important medical diagnoses and developmental history.

We may be assessing a child who has already been in the speech and language therapy system for a while and there already may be case notes available. In this case, the case history will be much shorter but is still necessary when a new therapist takes over.

The advantage of a face-to-face case history is that it is much easier to ask follow-up questions to seek further detail if an important factor has been raised. It is also a good opportunity to start building a relationship with the parents, who may be an integral part of the therapy process.

Although the case history interview is not usually a time to give parental advice, it may be appropriate to offer some helpful suggestions – especially if it seems that parents may need to adapt their way of responding to their child's speech difficulties more positively.

Parents may want answers, a diagnosis, or a prognosis at this early stage, but it is important not to feel pressured into making decisions too early. It is helpful to explain to parents that assessment is a process, and that this is just the initial information-gathering stage.

The following questions are useful in an initial case history interview, although the exact wording used will depend on the age of the child, the difficulties they present with, and whether they have already had therapy:

- 'What brought you here? What are your main concerns? Have you any thoughts on what the problem might be or thought of a "label"?'
- Other professionals: Has the child seen any other SALTs or other professionals? Is there an existing diagnosis?

- Family details: Parents, siblings, and extended family.
- Birth history: Any medical issues
- Early feeding skills: Issues with latching, chewing, gagging, swallowing, dealing with different textures, messy eating etc.
- Milestones: Age of crawling, walking, development of fine motor skills, general coordination.
- Social development: Interaction with peers, play skills, personality traits etc.
- Cognitive skills: Are any related concerns or reports available?
- Health issues: Illnesses, accidents, allergies, sleep and eating patterns, activity levels etc.
- Medical diagnoses: Are there any known diagnoses?
- Hearing history: Hearing test results, responses to sounds, history of upper respiratory tract infections etc.
- Intelligibility: What percentage can parents understand? How well do siblings, peers, other familiar/unfamiliar adults, and teachers understand? Does anyone 'interpret' for the child? Is intelligibility worse when the child is tired or unwell, or in longer utterances? How does intelligibility of single words compare with conversation?
- Babble: Extent of babbling, whether the child is unusually quiet, vocal play, vocalisations etc.
- Imitation: Tries to imitate often, makes little attempt to imitate, gets upset when asked to imitate, obviously struggles when trying to imitate.
- Sounds/words used: Age of first words, number of intelligible words currently used, whether words get 'lost' after being used for a while, other approximations of words used, willingness to copy or say words in different situations, volume of speech used.
- Languages spoken at home: Language(s) other than English used at home and whether the child uses words or phrases in the additional language(s). How does intelligibility vary with the language used?

- Expressive language (older children): Number of words used in a sentence, use of grammatically correct sentences, pronouns, verb tenses, question forms etc.
- Speech sounds: Which sounds are used/never used/sometimes used? Is there any struggle/mouthing of words/silent posturing?
- Consistency: Are sounds/words always produced in the same way or with variability?
- Non-speech oral skills: Blowing, sucking, blowing raspberries, imitating different faces, licking etc.
- Mode of communication: Use of gestures/signs/pulling/grunting instead of words or to support intelligibility.
- Frustration: Frustration when not understood, passivity, or unhappiness.
- Receptive language: Can the child understand spoken language in different environments? Are there any reported difficulties from nursery or school?
- Progress at school (older children): Progress with literacy, spelling, maths etc. What are teachers reporting? Does the child have appropriate attention and listening skills?
- Family history: Is there any history of speech disorder, dyslexia, coordination difficulties, or other developmental diagnoses?
- 'What advice have you been given from others? Are you trying any strategies or techniques? What has worked/not worked?'

With any child presenting with a possible SSD, questions relating to early sound production, feeding, babbling, and hearing are of particular importance.

Chapter 10

THE CORE SPEECH SAMPLE

WHAT IS THIS?

A core speech sample is the essential ingredient for all children with a suspected SSD, regardless of presentation. It is the starting point for further assessment and should signpost us to the areas we need to look at in more detail. Based on the findings of this initial assessment, further specific tests – such as those for inconsistency, articulation, phonology, and oromotor skills – can be carried out. 'Red flags' raised during the case history interview may also suggest the need for further assessment in specific areas.

The core speech sample may be taken at any point during the therapeutic process and can be used as a way of monitoring progress and making decisions such as when and whether to discharge.

The DEAP assessment is commonly used by SALTs as the initial screen and is the only standardised assessment used for SSDs, alongside the Toddler Phonology Test (TPT), designed to assess phonological acquisition in children aged between 2;0 and 2;11 years. The DEAP has been called the 'gold standard' assessment for SSDs by the RCSLT. However, other published assessments may also be used, as well as the therapist's own materials for eliciting a speech sample.

The core speech sample should always include the following:

- Single word production.
- Stimulability for C, CV, VC, and VCV.
- Connected speech.
- Consistency.

DOI: 10.4324/9781003480778-13

- Intelligibility rating.
- Subjective impressions of nasality, prosody, and other suprasegmental areas.

SINGLE WORD PRODUCTION

A small number of words can initially be used to get an idea of the child's production in single words. In the DEAP assessment, the initial screening assessment has ten pictures to name which include many, but not all, of the consonants and vowels in English in different word positions. The pictures are named and transcribed three times in total (following the instructions in the manual), which shows us how consistent the child is. For two-year olds, the TPT has 37 pictures to name, and error patterns are identified and analysed according to whether they are typical for the child's age, typical but delayed, or atypical. Other assessments commonly used include the South Tyneside Assessment of Phonology and the CLEAR Phonology Screening Assessment. Alternatively, therapists can use their own collection of objects or pictures to elicit a range of sounds in different syllable and word positions.

We can look for immediate signs of delayed phonological processes – such as fronting, stopping, or cluster reduction – or signs of distortion articulation disorder. We will not know whether a child has a substitution articulation disorder (ie, they are not producing specific sounds) until we have assessed their ability to produce these sounds in isolation or in other word positions.

Accurate transcription of the child's speech is essential and is covered in Section 12.

STIMULABILITY FOR C, CV, VC, AND VCV

If a child is not using a specific sound in single words, we then need to assess whether they can produce it in isolation on imitation and in CV, VC, and VCV positions. 'Stimulability' refers to whether the child can imitate the sound or syllable accurately, either by themselves or after modelling by the therapist. The therapist should not give too many cues, such as visual or verbal placement cues, during the assessment, as this constitutes 'therapy, and if the child produces the target sound accurately, this may be due to a 'therapeutic' effect. However, another type of assessment – *dynamic assessment* – does utilise this type of cueing and is discussed in Section 11. If the child can produce the target sound better with certain cues, this gives us valuable information as to the type of therapy cues to use during treatment. It also provides us with insight on how well the child can imitate, especially if CAS is suspected. Dynamic assessment can show up features such as groping which may not be evident in a straightforward picture-naming test.

If the child is *unable* to imitate the sound in isolation or *can* produce the sound in isolation but only in *one* vocalic context, (out of CV, VC, and VCV), it is an *articulatory* error. However, if the child *can* produce the sound in two or three vocalic contexts, it is a *phonological* error.

For example, if the child says 'sun' /sʌn/ → [dʌn] in a picture-naming assessment but can produce [s] in isolation spontaneously and can imitate /s/ correctly but not 'sea' /si/, the error is *articulatory*. If the child says 'sun' /sʌn/ → [dʌn] but then imitates 'sea' and 'mouse' correctly, the error is *phonological*.

This may seem a little complicated, but distinguishing between an *articulatory* and *phonological* error is probably the most important difference to establish in assessment, as this will dictate the type of therapy that is indicated.

CONNECTED SPEECH

It is important to assess this, so we can listen out for:

- Whether the child is generalising sounds into conversation.
- Their use of prosody, nasality, volume, rate, and other suprasegmental features.
- Their overall intelligibility.

We can elicit connected speech by carrying out a language assessment such as the Renfrew Action Picture Test (RAPT), which can also be used as a measure of the child's expressive language; or by asking them to describe a picture or talk about their family. With younger children, this can be done through informal play.

Transcription can be orthographic (written words), rather than phonemic, but it is important to listen out carefully for evidence of unusual features.

CONSISTENCY

This can be assessed by asking the child to rename the pictures again, preferably twice more, and comparing the productions each time. The DEAP has this element built into the screening test, but you can do this yourself using any suitable stimuli.

For a child to have a significant level of *inconsistency*, they need to have 40% or more inconsistency at the single-word level. If so, further assessment is needed to see whether they may have IPD or CAS.

INTELLIGIBILITY RATING

This can be assessed subjectively, in connected speech, as part of the initial assessment. We should make subjective ratings of overall intelligibility to unfamiliar listeners versus close family members and intelligibility on known versus unknown conversational topics.

One way of doing this quickly is by using a five-point rating scale for both a parent and an unfamiliar listener as follows:

1. Unintelligible in conversation.
2. Occasionally intelligible in conversation.
3. Often intelligible in conversation.
4. Mostly intelligible in conversation.
5. Completely intelligible in conversation.

Although this type of rating is unreliable, it is useful for comparing impressions of intelligibility in the same child over time and between 'raters'.

SUBJECTIVE IMPRESSIONS OF NASALITY, PROSODY, AND OTHER SUPRASEGMENTAL AREAS

These can be gathered during conversation or informal play with the child, or when the connected speech sample is being taken. It can be helpful to record the child's connected speech, as it can be hard to listen out for every aspect and write it down while the child is in front of you. Recording the child's speech is particularly useful for identifying more subtle features, particularly suprasegmental aspects of speech. Recordings can also be used to play (anonymously) to other SALTs, so that a second pair of ears – and someone unfamiliar with the child's speech – can objectively rate intelligibility or other features.

We should also listen out for anything unusual, such as hyponasality, hypernasality, flat or unusual intonation, irregular or unusual rate, volume, pitch, or voice quality.

USEFUL RESOURCES

CLEAR Phonology Screening Assessment. www.clear-resources.co.uk/AssessmentP1.html

Dodd et al (2012). DEAP. www.pearsonclinical.co.uk/store/ukassessments/en/Store/Professional-Assessments/Speech-%26-Language/Diagnostic-Evaluation-of-Articulation-and-Phonology/p/P100009266.html

McIntosh and Dodd (2011). Toddler Phonology Test (TPT). Pearson Assessment. www.pearsonclinical.co.uk/store/ukassessments/en/Store/Professional-Assessments/Speech-%26-Language/Toddler-Phonology-Test/p/P100009235.html

McLeod et al (2012). Intelligibility in Context Scale. www.csu.edu.au/research/multilingual-speech/ics

Renfrew (2019). *Action Picture Test* (5th edition). Routledge.

Winslow Resources. STAP 2. www.winslowresources.com/south-tyneside-assessment-of-phonology-2-stap-2.html

Chapter 11

DETAILED SPEECH ASSESSMENT

WHY MIGHT THIS BE NEEDED?

It may be clear to us that a child has a straightforward SSD involving, for example, one phonological process or one articulatory distortion, which we can start working on without the need for a more in-depth assessment. We do not want to spend time carrying out unnecessary assessments. However, where a child has a more complex presentation, we may need to carry out further in-depth analysis, and the results from the core speech sample should have highlighted areas for further assessment. Detailed assessment is likely to require more than one session to carry out.

Examples of why we might conduct more detailed assessment include the following:

- Where more detailed phonemic/phonetic transcription of a wider variety of words and syllable structures is needed to gain greater insight into the specific areas of difficulty.
- For the specific assessment of vowels, if there is evidence of distortion or substitution.
- For the assessment of polysyllabic words and/or clusters.
- For the further assessment of suprasegmental features such as nasality, prosody, voice etc.
- For the assessment of phonological awareness if there are concerns in this area, especially if literacy is an area of concern.
- Where a full oral examination and oromotor assessment are indicated.
- If the child's speech is complex and/or CAS is suspected.

DOI: 10.4324/9781003480778-14

HOW TO CARRY OUT A MORE DETAILED SPEECH ASSESSMENT

- Transcribe further words within the target areas which include target sounds in different phonetic contexts and word structures, and repeated productions of some words several times, to test for inconsistency. Five or more examples of a phonological process are needed before we can say that a child has that process in their sound system. The exception is for weak syllable deletion, for which only two examples are needed.
- Assess stimulability of sounds which are not produced accurately in words, both in isolation and in non-words. It is said to be 'stimulable' if it can be produced accurately in isolation and, in the case of a consonant, produced accurately in at least two syllable positions. Cues can be given (eg, verbal, visual, auditory) in the elicitation tasks.
- Record a longer speech sample and transcribe sections of this if possible (using orthographic, broad phonemic, or narrow phonetic transcription, as needed).

HOW TO ANALYSE THE SPEECH SAMPLE

The following areas should be analysed, unless a formal assessment has been used – such as the Nuffield Dyspraxia Programme Assessment (NDP3 Speech Assessment) or the DEAP – which provides its own scoring and analysis:

- Inventories:
  - Consonants.
  - Vowels.
  - Word structures (eg, CVs, CVCs, clusters).
- Processes and patterns:
  - Which phonological processes are present (age-appropriate, delayed, or atypical?)
  - Variability: Is there widespread unexplained variability? Is this context dependent or does it relate to how recently the words were acquired?

- What are the patterns of phoneme collapse? (This helps with choosing therapy targets and stimuli to use in therapy.)
- What word-level errors are present (eg, consonant harmony, sequencing errors, or consonant/vowel insertions)?
- What phonetic errors are present (eg, distortions of 's' or 'r', weakly articulated consonants, errors as a secondary consequence of hearing impairment, cleft palate, a developmental syndrome)?
- Are there phonetic errors present which are an intermediate stage before correct production is achieved (ie, the child is showing evidence of progression)?
- Are there vowel errors (either as a phonological process or as distortions in length etc)?
- What factors are affecting intelligibility? Is this mainly due to substitution errors? Are there distorted co-articulatory transitions across word boundaries or inappropriate use of pauses or glottal stops?
- Is the child using appropriate prosody?
- What is the percentage of consonants correct? This can indicate severity and is also used to monitor progress and as an outcome measure.

ADDITIONAL ASSESSMENTS

The following may also be needed, depending on the findings from the previous analysis:

- Stimulability assessment.
- Oromotor assessment.
- Inconsistency assessment.
- Psycholinguistic assessment.
- Intelligibility assessment.

USEFUL RESOURCES

Bates, S, Titterington, J and Child Speech Disorder Research Network, UK (2021). Good Practice Guidelines for the Analysis of Child Speech (2nd edition). Ulster University. https://pure.ulster.ac.uk/ws/portalfiles/portal/93134795/Good_practice_guidelines_for_the_analysis_of_child_speech_2nd_edition_2021.pdf

Chapter 12

TRANSCRIPTION

WHAT IS THIS USED FOR?

Transcription is a skill that SALTs are uniquely trained to do and is an essential part of taking and analysing a speech sample. Transcription aims to be an accurate, objective record of how a child is speaking and we cannot diagnose a speech disorder without it.

The main functions of transcription are as follows:

- To analyse the details of a child's speech patterns.
- To provide a permanent record of speech production at a specific point in time.
- To signpost us towards additional assessments that should be carried out.
- To aid differential diagnosis.
- As evidence to back up a diagnosis.
- To inform the decision on which therapy approach to use.
- To assist in target setting.
- To measure progress during therapy.
- To give concrete information to another therapist when a case changes hands.

TYPES OF TRANSCRIPTION

BROAD (PHONEMIC) TRANSCRIPTION

This uses phonetic symbols to transcribe the child's speech in terms of 'phones' and should include marking the primary stressed syllable with a dash (for words with two or more syllables). We use slant brackets for phonemic transcription.

This level of transcription is usually sufficient for most children; however, if there is a significant level of distortion, we may need to use more detail so that more subtle features can be captured and recorded. Examples might be in cases of hearing impairment, cleft palate, dysarthria, or CAS.

NARROW (PHONETIC) TRANSCRIPTION

This uses all segmental details with diacritics added to the symbols which give details about the child's realisation, such as degree of nasality, aspiration, and whether the vowel is too high (close) or too low (open). Square brackets are used for narrow transcription and primary stress and syllable markers are not included. There are many different diacritics available; however, although this skill is covered in SALT training courses, many qualified therapists do not use narrow transcription often enough to maintain the skills they learned during training. Others may not have had the opportunity to spend enough time during training to acquire a high skill level in this area.

IS IT ACCURATE?

Although transcription aims to be clear and unambiguous, it is not 100% accurate; but we should see it as a way of deciding whether a child's realisation is 'acceptable' or 'good enough'. If it is not, what does the child do instead? Broad phonemic transcription has been found to be fairly accurate between different raters, but narrow phonemic transcription varies considerably between raters. This is unsurprising, since there is such a wide variety of different diacritics which can be used and we each use our own perceptual skills to make decisions about tiny differences in the sound.

The main objective is to decide whether a sound is 'acceptable' and, if not, to make as accurate a record as possible about what the child is doing instead.

Each SALT will differ in their level of transcription skills, but it is possible to refine existing skills through training and practice. SALTs who work with certain groups of children, such as those with cleft palates, need a particularly advanced level of transcription skills. However, it is important that therapists working with a more general caseload have a sufficiently trained ear to be able to detect subtle differences in a child's speech that may indicate the need for further multidisciplinary assessment, particularly where a cleft palate is suspected.

SHOULD WE ALWAYS TRANSCRIBE?

It is important to have a permanent record of a child's speech sample, even if no SSD is detected. This will serve as evidence in the future if the parents query an SSD when the child is older. With very young children, it is vital to have some early evidence of their speech patterns so that their progress can be tracked. This should be done even if the child has a very small number of protowords or if the predominant focus of therapy is language development rather than speech.

The RCSLT Good Practice Guidelines for Transcription of Children's Speech Samples in Clinical Practice and Research (2017a) clearly set out the key role of transcription with SSDs and provide essential guidance for SALTs.

HOW TO TRANSCRIBE

- Aim for live transcription if possible and sit opposite the child, so that you have a clear view of their face and can spot key visual cues such as jaw slide, groping, asymmetry, silent articulations, and tongue and lip positions.
- Record the speech sample if possible, so that it can be listened to several times, as features such as nasality, prosody, schwa insertion, vowel distortion, and overall intelligibility may be easier to hear and analyse. Note that any recordings are part of the child's clinical records and parental consent is needed. Therapists should adhere to current RCSLT policies and those of their own organisation.
- Use symbols from the International Phonetic Alphabet chart and the extended International Phonetic Alphabet chart.

- Write the English word orthographically in inverted commas, followed by a broad transcription of the adult version in slant brackets. Include a dash to mark the primary stressed syllable and use vowels which reflect the child's local dialect, not the therapist's dialect, if there is a difference.
- Use an arrow from the adult version to the child's realisation of the word in slant brackets for phonemic transcription and square brackets for phonetic transcription. For phonemic transcription, include primary stress and syllable markers. For phonetic transcription, include as many diacritics as possible to describe the sound. If you can't remember or don't know the diacritic, a written description can be very helpful.
- Include the word structure of the target and the child's realisation (eg, CVC, CCVCC).
- Remember that there are, strictly speaking, no 'medial' consonants, as these are considered the first sound of the second syllable. For example, in the word 'weeny'/wi.ni/, the /n/ is the initial sound in the *second* syllable. It is described as a *within-word, syllable-initial* sound (WWSI).
- If there are consonant distortions, try to transcribe these phonetically, using diacritics to indicate features such as palatisation, dentalisation, or uvular articulation of velars. Articulation which is more 'forward' or 'backward' can also be indicated, as well as unreleased plosives, inadequate airflow, and weak articulation.
- Vowel distortions should be transcribed phonetically, according to the tongue and jaw position (the tongue may be too far back or forward, and the jaw may be too open or too closed). Vowel length may be unusual, and nasality and voice quality may also be different, so all these features should be indicated using diacritics.

Here are some examples of correct phonemic transcription:

- 'cluck' /klʌk/ CCVC → /kʌk/ CVC
- 'table' /ˈteɪ.bɔ/ CVCV → /ˈti.ti/ CVCV
- 'umbrella' /ʌm.ˈbɹe.lə/ VCCCVCV → /ˈbe.lə/ CVCV

WHAT COUNTS AS 'ACCEPTABLE'?

There is wide variation in how children produce sounds and we need to decide what is 'acceptable' and what is 'not acceptable'. If a child is using a sound which is part of their local dialect, such as a glottal stop word-finally in London, this is considered acceptable. We need to look at the child in the context of their environment, family, and peers to make these decisions. Realisation of vowels varies significantly depending on the geographical area, whether the child has English as an additional language (EAL), and the local dialect. Children with EAL may often use sounds which they also use in their home language, and these are perfectly acceptable and should never be considered 'errors'. We certainly don't want to spend precious time working on speech sounds which are acceptable in the child's family or community.

USEFUL RESOURCES

Child Speech Disorder Research Network (2017). Good practice guidelines for the transcription of children's speech in clinical practice and research. www.nbt.nhs.uk/sites/default/files/BSLTRU_Good%20practice%20guidelines_Transcription_2Ed_2017.pdf

Chapter 13

ORAL EXAMINATION/ OROMOTOR SCREEN

WHEN IS AN ORAL EXAMINATION NEEDED?

It may be inappropriate to carry out an oral examination on a young child during an initial assessment; in fact, this may scare off the child completely! However, there are times when an oral examination is particularly important as part of the diagnostic process. Here is when one is definitely needed, albeit not necessarily in the first session:

- When a child presents with an SSD with unusual speech features (eg, excessive hypo or hypernasality, or unusual sound substitutions).
- When the child appears to have an unusual facial appearance or dentition.
- If there appears to be significant congestion and the child appears to be a mouth-breather.
- If the parent reports concerns with feeding.
- Where a known structural difference is reported by the parents.

The purpose of the oral examination is to check for the presence of any unusual structural features that may contributing to or causing the speech problem, and to determine whether the child needs to be referred to another professional, such as an ear, nose and throat (ENT) consultant, a regional cleft palate team, or an orthodontist.

HOW TO CARRY OUT AN ORAL EXAMINATION

- Consider wearing personal protective equipment, including a high-quality facemask. This is particularly important for SALTs who are pregnant, as there are infections (eg, cytomegalovirus) which can be harmful to babies in utero.
- Adhere to strict handwashing protocol.
- Ensure that the parents have signed a consent form, and that the child has been given a verbal explanation about what to expect and has given their verbal consent.
- Ask the child to open their mouth really wide (perhaps use an analogy such as 'crocodile mouth') and encourage them to keep it open wide throughout.
- Use a torch and look carefully for the following features, perhaps using a spatula to keep the tongue down for a clearer view:
  - Check the dentition: Are the teeth aligned and are there any missing? Is there good dental hygiene?
  - Are the lips symmetrical and are there any unusual features?
  - Is the jaw symmetrical and correctly aligned?
  - Do the hard and soft palate appear normal? Is there a bifid uvula or any other unusual signs?
  - Does the tongue appear normal in terms of size, shape, and colour? Is there a tongue-tie (known as 'ankyloglossia')?
  - Are the tonsils enlarged or infected?

Key diagnostic features to look out for include the following:

- Signs of a submucous cleft: There may be a bifid uvula, a blue tinge, or a bump on the hard palate. If any of these is present, a referral to the regional cleft lip and palate team is necessary to rule out the presence of a submucous cleft.
- Enlarged tonsils: If there is also a history of recurrent upper respiratory tract infections, hyponasality, and snoring, the child should be referred to an ENT specialist and

for a hearing test. These factors mean that the child is at increased risk of hearing difficulties due to glue ear. Most surgeons are now reluctant to carry out adenoidectomies and tonsillectomies, or to insert grommets, unless there is a significant impact on the child's hearing. In the absence of a hearing difficulty, enlarged tonsils and adenoids can cause the child significant discomfort and can affect intelligibility if the enlargement is significant. The hope is that they will reduce in size over time and the impact may lessen as the child grows.

- Unusual dentition: An open bite (when there is a gap between the front top and bottom teeth when the child tries to close their teeth together) may indicate the prolonged use of a dummy or baby bottle or continual thumb-sucking. It may also occur with a tongue thrust. An open bite may cause speech difficulties and it is important that, if there is a known cause, this is reversed. In some cases, the open bite can resolve itself, but it may need orthodontic intervention if not. When the front teeth are missing in a young child (eg, due to accident or dental decay), this may cause speech difficulties – particularly an interdental lisp – as there is no natural 'barrier' to prevent the tongue from pushing forwards.
- Tongue-tie: The frenulum may be shorter, tightened, or thickened. Ways to spot this, if it is not otherwise obvious, include a heart-shaped tongue when it is pushed forward and an inability to curl the tongue towards the nose or lick around the lips. The frenulum can usually stretch as the child grows and is rarely a primary cause of SSDs. It may sometimes cause difficulties with articulation of specific sounds, such as /l/; however, it is more likely to affect feeding and good oral hygiene. Some parents feel that their child's speech difficulties will resolve if they have surgery on the tongue-tie; however, we cannot guarantee that a speech difficulty is directly due to a tongue-tie and trying therapy is always a good way to start.

WHEN SHOULD WE CARRY OUT AN OROMOTOR ASSESSMENT?

This should be carried out as part of a differential diagnosis where the child appears to have speech features such as inconsistency, restricted range and movement of articulators, or unusual nasality; where the child presents with a moderate to severe SSD; or where the parents report a known difficulty. An oromotor assessment is necessary to identify the presence of oral apraxia. It can identify difficulties with the speed, range, strength, and accuracy of muscle movements, and can help to differentiate between CAS and dysarthria. It is also necessary to look at potential structural abnormalities or differences such as submucus cleft palate or velopharyngeal insufficiency.

HOW TO CARRY OUT AN OROMOTOR ASSESSMENT

There are two oromotor assessment formats which are commonly used by SALTs:

- The DEAP has a quick screening assessment which covers DDK sequencing, intelligibility and fluency, isolated movements of tongue and lips, and sequenced movements. The child is scored on a scale of 0-3, according to accuracy. This is a very useful screen to establish whether more detailed assessment is needed.
- The NDP3 is much more detailed and covers the areas of lips and jaw, airstream, voice, palate, and tongue. This is useful if a degree of oromotor difficulty has already been identified.

A therapist may also choose to carry out their own informal oromotor screening assessment. The three main areas which are important to assess are isolated movements, movement sequences, and DDK. The child should be given a demonstration of the required movement to imitate, as listed below:

- Isolated movements (note anything unusual in terms of speed, accuracy, symmetry, or other associated movements):
  - Lips: Open/closed/spread/pursed (also note reported difficulties with feeding or dribbling).
  - Tongue: Out of mouth/into mouth, up to top lip/down towards chin, movement to one side/other side (also note reported difficulties with dribbling, licking, and chewing).
- Movement sequences (note speed, accuracy, symmetry, or other associated movements):
  - Tongue out, then blow.
  - Open mouth, then close and smile.
  - Tongue to top lip, then purse lips.
- DDK (note accuracy, speed, signs of struggle, and inconsistency): Ask the child to repeat the following ten times:
  - 'Buttercup.'
  - 'Pat-a-cake.'
  - 'Caterpillar.'

Any difficulties with the above areas should be assessed in more detail, perhaps using the NDP3.

The findings of the oral examination and oromotor assessment should be used, alongside the speech assessment findings and case history information, to help make a differential diagnosis. This may also involve referral to another agency (eg, audiology, paediatrician, regional cleft palate team, orthodontist), depending on the findings.

REFERENCES

Dodd et al (2012). DEAP. www.pearsonclinical.co.uk/store/ukassessments/en/Store/Professional-Assessments/Speech-%26-Language/Diagnostic-Evaluation-of-Articulation-and-Phonology/p/P100009266.html

Nuffield Centre Dyspraxia Programme Ltd. NDP3 (Nuffield Dyspraxia Programme Speech Assessment). www.ndp3.org

Chapter 14

THE PRE-VERBAL CHILD

Children who have no or very little spoken output present a diagnostic challenge to SALTs. Parents are often desperate to understand why their child is not yet talking, but it is important to avoid making suggestions about a possible SSD at this stage when the child is presenting with an expressive language delay.

WHY MIGHT A CHILD HAVE NO VERBAL OUTPUT?

As we know, the reasons why a child may have no or very little spoken output for their age are numerous and include the following:

- Fluctuating hearing loss (due to glue ear).
- Selective mutism.
- ASD.
- Global developmental delay.
- Environmental reasons (eg, reduced opportunity or need to communicate verbally).
- A specific speech disorder such as CAS
- Expressive language delay with no obvious cause.
- Developmental language disorder (DLD)

Most children who present to SALTs as pre-verbal do develop spoken language appropriately in time; however, we need to be aware of some 'at-risk' factors that may lead us to think that the child may be more likely to have an SSD, even though it is not possible to diagnose this until the child has developed more spoken language. The symptom cluster of a child with a speech disorder will change over time: the child may present with expressive language delay, but as they start using more words, the disordered features of speech may become apparent.

'AT-RISK' FACTORS FOR SSDS

FEEDING

In the case history interview, the parents may have mentioned difficulties with feeding, sucking, and chewing; or other oromotor issues, such as excessive dribbling. If feeding difficulties are ongoing, it is important that the child is referred to an ENT specialist to rule out the possibility of an undiagnosed cleft palate, particularly if there is nasal regurgitation. Any swallowing difficulties should always be referred as a matter of urgency to a SALT who specialises in this area.

A small proportion of children with a history of feeding, sucking, and chewing difficulties go on to have a diagnosis of CAS; although feeding difficulties are a feature of oromotor dyspraxia rather than CAS, the two may co-occur.

Parents may mention concerns about tongue-tie, which may have been picked up at or soon after birth, especially if the baby has had difficulty latching on at the breast. There is little evidence that tongue-tie adversely affects speech development, so it is not a significant predictive factor for SSDs.

HISTORY OF HEARING PROBLEMS

If there have been known hearing problems from a young age and the child is pre-verbal, they are certainly at risk of an SSD. Where the child has glue ear, the earlier this is present, the more likely it is that their speech and language development will be significantly affected. Babies with glue ear in the first six months of life often have severely delayed and disordered speech sound development, as well as significant language delay. Children with moderate or severe sensorineural hearing loss from birth are likely to develop speech and language differently as compared to hearing children, and the support of a specialist SALT and a multidisciplinary team will be needed to coordinate holistic assistance for the child and their family.

DELAYED EXPRESSIVE LANGUAGE DEVELOPMENT

Many children who have SSDs have a history of expressive language delay, although this alone is not diagnostic.

LACK OF OR REDUCED BABBLING

Children who don't babble or have limited babbling are at greater risk of SSDs. Children with CAS often have a history or no or little babbling, and often exhibit marked differences in both the quantity and quality of their babbling, which may have very few syllable strings (eg, 'mamamama', 'dadadada' and strings in which the vowel changes, such as 'beeboobeeboo'). Parents of children with CAS may report sounds such as grunts and squeals rather than these varied syllable strings. Again, this is also reported in children with hearing loss. Children with severe CAS may also appear to be struggling to vocalise at all and may show signs of struggle when trying to imitate.

FAMILY HISTORY

There is some evidence that SSDs may run in families, although the presentation may not be identical in all family members affected. Family history is not diagnostic in itself but should be noted.

DIFFICULTIES IN PRODUCING SPEECH

Parents may report that their child has intent to communicate but shows signs of struggle when trying to imitate sounds or syllables. They may produce a limited range of sounds and syllable structures. Children who are diagnosed later with CAS may have these features in their early speech and, in severe cases, may exhibit visible 'groping' or struggle when attempting to imitate. Children with other types of SSDs may also use a limited range of sounds and atypical phonological patterns.

'AT-RISK' FACTORS FOR PERSISTENT SSD

The following factors have been identified in the literature as significant risk factors for persistent SSD and are thus useful when making clinical prioritisation decisions for early intervention for SSDs.

The figures in brackets below indicate the degree of increased risk of PSSD: 100% is equivalent to doubling the risk. A combination of factors is likely to increase the total risk compared with the presence of just one or two factors:

- Low socioeconomic status (50%).
- Unintelligible to strangers at age three years (140%).
- Not combining words at age two years (80%).
- History of weak sucking at four weeks (40%).
- Poor with word morphology at age three years (unquantified).
- Patterns of speech disorder rather than delay at age four years (100%).
- More likely to be reported as having had coordination problems before age eight years (100%).
- More likely to have had grommets or hearing impairment before age eight years (100%).
- More likely to struggle with nonword repetition (unquantified).

(RCSLT, 2019)

ASSESSING A PRE-VERBAL CHILD

A pre-verbal child should be assessed with no preconceptions as to the reasons why. All areas of development should be looked at, including motor development, social interaction and communication, play skills, and verbal comprehension, as well as a full case history. Time should be spent with the parents to see how they are interacting with their child and providing an environment in which the child can develop spoken language.

Sometimes parents use the term 'non-verbal' or 'pre-verbal' to mean that their child is using words which are not recognisable or not produced in the adult form. If this is the case, it is important to be very positive and help the parents to understand the significance of their child using words to communicate, even if their realisation of those words is not yet accurate.

At this stage, any sounds or words used by the child should be listened to carefully and transcribed as best as possible. It is important to look at the range of vowels and consonants used, babble sequences, the ability to imitate accurately, and the use of CV, VC, CVC, or more complex phonotactic structures. Also listen out for non-segmental features such as nasality, resonance, voice, and intonation. For example, a child may reportedly be 'non-verbal'; but when observed, they may be using appropriate intonation for short phrases – such as 'ready, steady, go' – without any recognisable consonants being used.

Also look for signs of attempted sound or word formation by the child. A child who has the desire to speak but has severe CAS may show visible signs of trying to vocalise or move their mouth into the correct position, even if no sound comes out. They may also try to use other means of communication spontaneously, such as their own gestures, alongside pointing. Analysis of videos which parents have made at home are valuable for assessment of communication with us as observers. It is possible to spot aspects of speech production and communication which may be missed in a one-off face-to-face assessment.

If a child uses no spoken words, the assessment should focus on establishing the level of verbal comprehension (using formal and informal means), analysing social communication and play, and identifying the communication modalities used (eg, pulling, pointing, signing, gesture, grunting, crying). Even where no actual words are used, we can still listen out for sounds and intonation patterns as a baseline against which to monitor changes over time.

REFERENCES

RCSLT (2019). Child speech sound disorder: special edition. www.rcslt.org/wp-content/uploads/media/Project/Bulletins/bulletin-august-ask-the-experts.pdf

Chapter 15

ASSESSING THE IMPACT ON THE CHILD'S ACTIVITY AND PARTICIPATION

SSDS AND THE WIDER CONTEXT

Any SSD, regardless of severity, may affect how the child interacts with the people around them and how confident they are as communicators, among other factors. There are also many factors which SALTs should consider when assessing and treating children with SSDs, which don't show up in assessments that focus solely on speech and language functioning.

The WHO developed a classification to support health and wellness known as the International Classification of Functioning, Disability and Health – Children and Youth (ICF-CY), which can be applied to children with SSDs in the following areas.

BODY STRUCTURE

Children who have an altered physical appearance related to a structural difference may have a reduced or altered ability to participate fully in society. Examples include cases of cleft lip and/or palate, developmental or acquired neurological disorders such as cerebral palsy or stroke, orofacial myofunctional disorders, and significant dental malocclusions. Children may experience difficulties with participating fully in clubs and activities, and with fully engaging with friendship groups at school or outside school.

SALTs need to assess how an altered body structure in a child with an SSD affects their social participation and activities, and then take this into account when assessing, setting targets, carrying out therapy, and measuring outcomes.

Case example

Millie had an intrauterine stroke which resulted in dysarthria and CAS. Although she could walk unaided, she had a left-sided hemiplegia and dribbled significantly. She was very aware of her mobility limitations and dribbling, which caused her anxiety, especially when meeting new children or teachers at school. Although assessment primarily highlighted her dysarthria and CAS, it also considered the effect of her altered body structure on her ability to communicate effectively and confidently with peers and adults. Therapy goals included Millie's ability to initiate conversation with peers and ongoing assessment of this area of communication was an important factor in measuring therapy outcomes.

BODY FUNCTION

The ICF-CY includes functions such as articulation, voice, fluency, hearing, breathing, and intellectual and mental functions such as temperament and personality. Speech production is integral to or significantly affected by these factors, and the areas of personality and temperament are especially important to include when assessing, setting targets, and choosing a therapy approach.

Case example

Jake presented with a severe SSD with features of inconsistent phonological disorder. Although he was highly unintelligible at age three and a half and was a high priority for direct speech and language therapy, there were aspects of his personality and temperament which significantly affected his ability to access direct therapy at that time. He was extremely socially and communicatively withdrawn, and his mother reported that each of her three children had similar personality types, as did their father. It was unclear as to how much of Jake's temperament was related to the secondary effects of his SSD; however, this was a significant aspect of assessment and therapy planning. The SALT decided to spend some time working with the parents and carried out some non-directive play therapy with Jake until he was able to engage actively in therapy for his SSD.

ACTIVITIES AND PARTICIPATION

This involves assessment of a child's social life, interests, and, in the case of teenagers and older children, their ability to engage with work experience, voluntary work, and other areas that involve communication.

CASE EXAMPLE

Shay was 17 years old and wanted to apply to study medicine. He sought therapy for a pronounced interdental lisp, as he was concerned that this might disadvantage him in interviews, which was causing him a high level of anxiety. Assessment addressed not only speech-related factors but also his confidence levels in applying for and attending university interviews.

ENVIRONMENTAL FACTORS

The ICF-CY includes products and technology, support, relationships, and attitudes as environmental factors.

The role of the family is crucial when a child has an SSD, and parenting style and attitudes can have a profound effect on progress in therapy and emotional factors within the child. The assessment should explore the parents' attitudes, beliefs, and ways of responding to their child's speech. These may vary from lack of concern to excessive anxiety or criticism. Parenting style and attitudes are important in assessment, as a considerable amount of work may need to be done with the parents in terms of helping them to develop a positive and enabling attitude towards their child's speech – supporting, encouraging, practising at home with the appropriate intensity, and understanding that they are an integral part of the therapeutic process.

Other relevant environmental factors include socio-economic factors, such as a child's access to relevant technology, a variety of toys, opportunities to participate in clubs and other activities, and private speech and language therapy, if adequate National Health Service (NHS) therapy is unavailable.

PERSONAL FACTORS

Relevant factors for health and wellness in the ICF-CY include age, gender, race, other health conditions, coping styles, overall behaviour pattern, and character style. These factors should all be assessed and considered throughout the therapeutic process.

CASE EXAMPLE

Jude was diagnosed with consistent phonological disorder at age four. However, he was also going through diagnostic assessments for a severe form of epilepsy and had several hospital admissions as a result of seizures within a month. During this time, it was felt that Jude's other health needs were of primary importance and his parents were unable to manage attending sessions to work on speech until his epilepsy was under better control. Jude's condition stabilised and he was able to access speech and language therapy input several months later, which was successful.

These five components of the ICF-CY all interact, and by considering each in turn, we can view the child in their wider context rather than through the narrow lens of how they present in a clinical setting. Our goals, therapeutic interventions, and outcome measures can thus be adapted accordingly. The factors described above show how a child's SSD can have a knock-on effect on other aspects of their development; and conversely, these factors can also affect the child's SSD.

REFERENCE

WHO (2007). *International Classification of Functioning, Disability and Health – Version for Children and Youth: 2013-CY.* World Health Organization.

Chapter 16

ASSESSING NON-SPEECH AREAS

HOW TO DO THIS

As for all children referred with a concern about a communication impairment, each child must be assessed in areas other than speech. Even if the child presents with an obvious SSD, additional areas are often affected. Parents may focus on just the speech issue, as this may be the most obvious thing they have noticed, but if there is a significant language deficit also, this may need addressing first. Expressive language delay is common in children with SSDs, but there may be other areas of communication which are affected, either as an additional but unrelated area of difficulty or as a co-occurring feature of the SSD.

The areas we should look at depend on the age of the child, presenting or reported concerns, and issues raised during the case history interview and following subjective observation by the therapist. A balance must be struck between skimping on valuable assessment time and over-assessing, which eats into time that could be spent on therapy or with another child. Some assessments are very lengthy and it may be that at the outset, this level of detail is not needed before getting started on some therapy. It may take a while for a newly qualified therapist to learn how to strike this balance, but they will hone this skill as they gain experience.

An initial screening assessment of other areas of communication is recommended, so that we know which areas need more detailed assessment.

RECEPTIVE LANGUAGE

For younger children, this involves observation of their responses to questions or simple instructions in an informal play situation. Asking parents and nursery staff whether the child follows simple instructions is also important. Informal assessment of verbal comprehension of prepositions (eg, in/on/under) and big/little concepts is also easy using a selection of toys; and receptive vocabulary can be assessed informally using pictures or objects.

For older children, this involves more structured comprehension screening, such as using one, two, three, and four-keyword tasks. This can be conducted using the Derbyshire Language Scheme or an informal version of this, with a variety of objects and instructions presented at a variety of levels.

Informal comprehension screening, looking at the number of keywords that a child can follow, should include several options from which the child can choose. For example, to be a true two-word level instruction, 'Put the cat on the chair' would need other animals/objects that could be placed on the chair, as well as other places on which the cat could be placed (eg, a table and a box). To step this up to a three-word level instruction, another element would have to be introduced – for example, the option of putting it 'on', 'in' or 'under' – or a variety of different colours or sizes of objects presented.

It may also be useful to carry out one or two subtests from the Pre-school Clinical Evaluation of Language Fundamentals (CELF-2) or the CELF-5 to get an idea of where the child is at with understanding spoken language. If it appears that receptive language is an area of difficulty, the full assessment can be administered. Other helpful standardised assessments include the Test for Reception of Grammar (TROG-2) and the British Picture Vocabulary Scale (BPVS).

It is also important to look at other aspects of verbal comprehension, such as the child's ability to understand 'who', 'where', 'why', 'when' and 'how' questions, as well as concepts such as size, colour, shape, and prepositions. Other areas to assess, particularly with older children, include the ability to understand more abstract questions which involve prediction (eg, 'What might happen next?') and inference (eg, 'I wonder what she might be thinking?' or 'How do you know that he is sad?'). The Blank Levels of Questioning (sometimes known as the Language of Learning Model) is a helpful way of assessing a child's ability to reason and understand abstract language skills and various resources are available to help assess these skills in a child (see the references at the end of this section). These areas of receptive language can be screened informally by using pictures of different scenarios and asking a series of carefully chosen questions to see how well the child responds.

EXPRESSIVE LANGUAGE

For younger children, taking a language sample during play can give an idea of whether they are at a single-word level or above. Asking parents and nursery staff to give examples of the child's utterances is also valuable. If the child uses a mixture of words, signs, gestures, and other non-verbal means of communication, these should be included when recording the language sample, with clear reference to the mode of communication used. A video recording of the child communicating is very helpful, particularly for children who use different modes of communication.

For older children, transcribing some conversation orthographically is the best way to get an idea of a child's expressive language skills. The RAPT is also a quick and easy way of assessing expressive language and is a standardised test. The CELF-5 has several different subtests on expressive language and one or two of these can be administered as a screening test, followed by further subtests if some areas of difficulty are observed.

LISTENING AND ATTENTION

If the child appears to have difficulties in listening or focusing during the assessment, or if this has been raised as an area of concern, further time can be given to discussing this in more detail with parents and nursery/school.

IMAGINATIVE PLAY

Observe how the child plays with cars/trains/animals/dolls etc. Imaginative play in younger children can be assessed informally through observation or by using a more structured assessment, such as the Symbolic Play Test.

SOCIAL INTERACTION

Observe how the child interacts during the assessment and ask whether parents/school have any concerns regarding social interactions with adults or peers. If there are difficulties in this area, further assessment can be carried out; the Pragmatics Profile – a rating scale to be completed by a parent/carer or other professional – is a useful tool for this.

It is important to clarify whether any issues with social interaction are characteristic of a specific social communication difficulty in addition to the SSD, or whether the features present are due to the negative consequences of having an SSD (eg, reluctance to speak to peers or poor eye contact due to feeling self-conscious or experiencing communicative breakdown).

PHONOLOGICAL AWARENESS

For younger children, some informal assessment of this can be incorporated into the initial assessment by asking the child to clap out syllables in words of two syllables or more and then, depending on their age, asking them to identify initial sounds in a selection of CVC words – for example, by asking, 'What's the first sound in "bus"?' It is important that this is done in a way which relies not on letter knowledge, but purely on the child's auditory perception, discrimination, and ability to segment the word into phonemic units.

When children start school at age four or five, they should be able to segment words into syllables and to begin identifying initial sounds, then final sounds, in simple words. Children who have not yet developed awareness of syllables by the time they start school will not be ready for the demands of 'phonics' at school, which is a phoneme-level skill. This ability to detect syllable boundaries precedes the skill of detecting phoneme boundaries and identifying which phoneme comes where in a word. These phoneme-level skills are essential for literacy development and children are at risk of significant literacy difficulties if they are delayed in these skills. Awareness of rhyme is an important process in the development of literacy; however, this is not as important in the development of speech and is thus not an essential area to assess, unless there are literacy concerns.

If phonological awareness appears to be an area of difficulty for the child, or if literacy difficulties are reported alongside an SSD, the Newcastle Assessment of Phonological Awareness (NAPA) may be carried out. This is a dynamic, criterion-referenced assessment of phonological awareness, with low memory and language load. The NAPA looks at the child's ability to segment syllables, identify word-initial and word-final phonemes, and then manipulate these in more complex ways. This includes deleting and substituting phonemes in different auditory tasks (ie, not using written letters at all).

Other assessments of phonological awareness include subtests in the DEAP and CELF-5, as well as some specific assessments such as the Pre-School and Primary Inventory of Phonological Awareness (PIPA) and the Phonological Assessment Battery (PHAB).

MOTOR DEVELOPMENT

This can be observed informally, in addition to asking for information from parents/teachers/nursery staff. Poor motor coordination, although not diagnostic, can be associated with CAS, and is thus important to note during assessment.

COGNITIVE DEVELOPMENT

There may be a known cognitive delay in some younger children, or concerns may have been raised by parents and/or nursery teachers about a younger child's global development. If not, any signs of delays in other areas of development should be noted by the SALT.

The academic progress of older children at school is an indication of whether there may be any additional difficulties with literacy or overall cognitive development. If the child is significantly behind at school, more information can be gathered from teachers and parents, and it may be appropriate to recommend further assessment by an educational psychologist.

USEFUL PUBLISHED ASSESSMENTS

- BPVS (British Picture Vocabulary Scale): www.gl-assessment.co.uk/assessments/products/british-picture-vocabulary-scale/
- CELF-5 UK (Clinical Evaluation of Language Fundamentals): www.pearsonclinical.co.uk/store/ukassessments/en/celf-5-record-forms/Clinical-Evaluation-of-Language-Fundamentals-%7C-Fifth-Edition-Metalinguistics/p/P100009108.html
- CELF-Preschool: 3 UK: www.pearsonclinical.co.uk/store/ukassessments/en/Store/Professional-Assessments/Developmental-Early-Childhood/Clinical-Evaluation-of-Language-Fundamentals-Preschool-3-UK/p/P100072000.html
- DLS (Derbyshire Language Scheme): www.derbyshire-language-scheme.co.uk
- NAPA (Newcastle Assessment of Phonological Awareness): https://research.ncl.ac.uk/phonologicalawareness/assessmentandintervention/aboutthenapa/
- PHAB (Phonological Assessment Battery): www.gl-assessment.co.uk/assessments/products/phab2/
- PIPA (Preschool and Primary Inventory of Phonological Awareness): www.pearsonclinical.co.uk/store/ukassessments/en/Store/Professional-Assessments/Speech-%26-Language/Preschool-and-Primary-Inventory-of-Phonological-Awareness/p/P100009225.html
- RAPT (Renfrew Action Picture Test): www.routledge.com/Action-Picture-Test/Speechmark-Renfrew/p/book/9781138586208?srsltid=AfmBOoqh03MgJz1s9YdPAhU6FD_yABFXwYD2OB7UBfNkmH8-Ez80lTpK

- Symbolic Play Test: www.gl-assessment.co.uk/assessments/products/symbolic-play-test/
- TROG-2 (Test for Reception of Grammar): www.pearson-clinical.co.uk/store/ukassessments/en/Store/Professional-Assessments/Speech-%26-Language/Vocabulary/Test-for-Reception-of-Grammar/p/P100009232.html

USEFUL RESOURCES

Blank Levels of Questioning: Activities for assessment and therapy. www.twinkl.co.uk/teaching-wiki/blanks-levels-of-questioning

Chapter 17

THE CASE PROFILE AND DIAGNOSTIC STATEMENT

HOW TO SUMMARISE THE ASSESSMENT INFORMATION IN A CASE PROFILE

Depending on how complex the child's communication disorder is and how many areas are affected, extensive information may be collected from different sources which must be analysed and collated into summary format. This can then be used in a detailed written report, in a summary for parents and others, or for the therapist's own case notes. This case profile may subsequently be used as evidence to back up a diagnosis and to assist in making decisions about therapeutic intervention and targets.

Where an SSD is a child's primary area of need, the case profile may include the following, although not all of these areas may be relevant to each case:

- The child's strengths and weaknesses at the each of the following levels:
  - Single sounds.
  - CVs and VCs.
  - CVCs.
  - CVCVs.
  - Clusters.
  - Polysyllabic words.
  - Phrases and connected speech.
- Prosody, voice, and other suprasegmental features.
- Intelligibility.
- An indication of severity.

- Receptive and expressive language.
- Other affected areas (eg, listening skills, social communication, phonological awareness).

A NOTE ABOUT SEVERITY...

'Severity' is not formally defined in the literature, although it is something that parents frequently ask about and it does give them an idea of the extent to which an SSD may impact on their child's ability to communicate.

Care should be taken when using terms such as 'mild', 'moderate', and 'severe', as these may mean different things to different people (ie, they can be very ambiguous), and they are not static in nature. For example, a child who may present at age three with 'severe CAS' may not be considered to have 'severe CAS' a year later after receiving therapy. We can qualify any term we use to refer to severity to parents and others by describing the child's overall intelligibility, how much their speech differs from that expected for a child of their age in terms of number of speech sounds used or number of phonological processes present etc. It is also important to explain to parents that severity cannot be measured on a single parameter, and that other aspects of communication – such as communicative confidence – are equally important.

CASE EXAMPLES

Four-year-old Sofia has an SSD which could be described as 'severe' using speech measures only. However, she is a highly sociable and communicatively confident child who does not allow her poor intelligibility to impact on her sociability, and she uses every available way to get her message across.

Twelve-year-old George has an SSD which could be described as a 'mild' articulation disorder, affecting his articulation of 's'. He is fully intelligible, but the effect on his self-esteem and ability to socialise with his peers is significant.

These examples emphasise that severity terms should be used to describe not only the speech aspects, but also the impact on the child.

IS A DIAGNOSTIC LABEL NECESSARY?

Following on from earlier chapters about classification and the challenges in agreeing about how to label a child's SSD, we need to decide whether and how to assign a diagnostic label and how valuable this is. 'Labelling' a child can have negative connotations and parents may have strong opinions about this, worrying that their child may be on the receiving end of negative comments from peers or preconceived ideas from teachers at school. Parents may also be concerned about their child's own feelings about themselves. This is particularly relevant in the case of ASD, attention deficit hyperactivity disorder (ADHD), or dyslexia, where parents may be reluctant to have a 'label' assigned to their child too early on – partly because this is likely to be a lifelong diagnosis and perhaps due to a fear that the professionals may have been mistaken and misdiagnosed their child.

In the field of SSDs, there have historically been periods when SALTs were encouraged to *describe* the disordered speech features rather than 'label' the disorder. However, I would strongly emphasise the value of a firm diagnostic label or labels for SSDs, for the following reasons:

- The SALT can have clarity in their mind as to the precise nature of the speech breakdown.
- The appropriate therapeutic approach can be selected which specifically targets a breakdown at that level (eg, phonological versus articulatory versus a combination).
- Parents and other professionals can understand the nature of the SSD and are more likely to be fully on board with a therapeutic plan which is built on a sound initial diagnosis.

WHEN THERE IS NO CLEAR DIAGNOSIS

After a period of assessment (which may take anything from one to several sessions), we should have built up a case profile of the child and know which areas are affected and which may need ongoing investigation.

Sometimes the diagnosis is very clear and the child may fall neatly into one main subtype according to the DEAP classification. However, often this is not the case and the child may fall within several subtypes, perhaps with one being dominant.

For other children, we may still have a very unclear picture of their diagnosis despite having carried out a detailed assessment. It may be that the child is not yet old enough or may not yet have enough spoken output for us to give a firm diagnosis. In these cases, we can describe the features present and give a tentative diagnosis based on this, with a description of why. Our diagnosis is thus a working hypothesis and once therapy is underway, the picture may become clearer.

CAN WE CHANGE A DIAGNOSIS?

Sometimes our original diagnosis may change in response to new information which comes to light during therapy. Even if we made a confident diagnosis early on, a child's response to therapy can show us that our original decision may need to change – especially if the child does not respond to the type of therapy which should be effective for that type of SSD.

Also, the diagnosis may change as the child progresses through therapy – not because we were wrong initially, but because therapy has altered the nature of the disorder (which is ultimately diagnosed based on the speech characteristics that we hear). Differential diagnosis should thus be seen as an ongoing rather than one-off process.

CASE EXAMPLES

Jonah was assessed at age three years and ten months and was diagnosed with phonological delay, as he was using several immature processes (fronting of velars and stopping of all fricatives in all word positions). Phonological-based therapy resulted in him developing the plosive/fricative contrast consistently, and some phonological awareness intervention helped to develop his awareness of initial and final alveolars/velars in words. However, it became clear that he was consistently unable to produce velar consonants in CV and VC position on imitation, even though he knew where those sounds should be in words, which was the cause of some frustration for him. These sounds could be produced in isolation. The therapist changed the diagnosis to articulation disorder and therapy focused on the production of velar consonants, using an articulatory approach rather than a phonological one. Jonah progressed well with this approach and as soon as he had developed the production of velars in CV and VC positions, he rapidly started generalising them into conversation without any alveolar/velar substitution errors.

Jamal presented at age three years, nine months with significant features of CAS and was given a firm diagnosis of CAS with some immature phonological processes. Intensive therapy which focused on the CAS aspects of his speech had positive results and after two years, he no longer had significant CAS features; however, he had some residual phonological processes which had not resolved. His diagnosis was changed to that of phonological delay, as he no longer met any of the criteria for a CAS diagnosis. His therapy intervention changed to having a phonological basis in light of this.

THE DIAGNOSTIC STATEMENT

This is a brief, clear description of what the therapist believes is at the heart of the child's speech sound difficulties, which reflects the clinical thinking behind the diagnosis. It should illustrate the overlapping nature of presenting deficits and should include a statement of severity and prognosis. It may also contain a statement which rules out a particular disorder – for example, it may include the statement: '… shows no evidence of CAS.'

The diagnostic statement is key in communicating to parents and other professionals about the child's underlying disorder. More detail can be provided in a full written report, but this statement should contain the main facts.

These clear, unambiguous statements are particularly powerful when an application is being made for an Education, Health, and Care Plan (EHCP), or for other kinds of additional funding application to support a child with an SSD. This may be for a place in a specialist provision, for speech and language therapy provision in a mainstream class, or for teaching assistant support in class.

The diagnostic statement may need further explanation to be given verbally to clarify what the diagnosis means and the implications for the child. Parents are often very keen to know what the prognosis is for change and whether there may be long-term consequences for the child as a result of their SSD.

EXAMPLES OF A DIAGNOSTIC STATEMENT

Example 1

X has age-appropriate receptive and expressive language skills, social communication, and attention skills. She has a slowed rate of speech and more difficulties with accurate production of longer words and phrases than shorter single words. She has inconsistent speech errors – including vowel distortions and the addition of a schwa at the ends of words, alongside a tendency to segment words into individual syllables when speaking – and intonation is unusual. Speech is, however, fully intelligible in all contexts. These speech features are evidence to support a diagnosis of mild CAS (childhood apraxia of speech). She also has some additional delayed phonological processes which do not affect intelligibility significantly.

Given that X has no additional difficulties with cognition or other co-occurring developmental disorders, she is likely to make progress with these areas of speech with appropriate direct speech and language therapy intervention.

Example 2

Y has age-appropriate development in all areas other than speech. He has a delayed speech pattern which can be described as 'phonological delay': he consistently substitutes 's' for 'd' at the beginning of words, although 's' can be produced in single words on imitation. This sound substitution is known as 'stopping' and is a common sound substitution in the speech of younger children. All other sounds are produced appropriately for his age. Given the appropriate type of therapy, he is likely to make progress and develop this sound contrast fully.

Chapter 18

COMMUNICATING WITH OTHERS

This is one of the most important areas, apart from the actual therapy itself, which dictates how effective our intervention will be. We need to choose the best way for this communication to happen if it cannot be in person, and it works best to ask the other people involved which mode is best for them. The main people we are likely to be communicating with are as follows.

PARENTS

Parents are usually, but not always, our main point of contact in the therapeutic process. Our relationship with parents, from the point of referral to the point of discharge, is key to successful therapy. Our role with parents can include reassuring, encouraging, empowering, training, demonstrating, modelling, informing, teaching, and understanding. In the early years, the parents may be the ones who implement the therapy on a day-to-day basis, and building a relationship of trust is essential so that they are more likely to respond to our suggestions and advice. An understanding of the type of SSD, the possible reasons for it, and the rationale for our choice of therapy is key for parents to play a full, effective role in the therapeutic process. It can help to prevent them from giving unhelpful verbal cues to their child at home and from trying their own interventions, which may be working against what we are trying to achieve. Parents have a unique role to play, in that they usually have that daily contact with the child which SALTs do not have, so they can implement strategies daily and monitor change frequently. Time invested in working with parents is time well spent.

OTHER FAMILY MEMBERS AND CARERS

Grandparents, other family members, or carers may be the people who bring the child to therapy sessions regularly, and any follow-up work which we expect families to carry out should be feasible and realistic for the individuals who are being asked to do the activities. Where possible, we should send follow-up work through to the parents and other adults who are responsible for carrying it out.

SCHOOLS/NURSERIES

Fostering good working relationships with the schools in which we work has a knock-on effect on the success of our therapy. Schools need to know that we have the knowledge, skills, and expertise to make the recommendations that we do. By taking a little extra time to explain, demonstrate, and suggest resources to use, we can greatly influence the level of support that teaching assistants can provide to our children.

It can also be helpful to involve schools in our goal-setting process, as there may be areas of communication which a child's teacher is concerned about in the classroom, but which we have not included in our goals.

OTHER SALTS

Working with other SALTs can be highly effective, provided that we communicate regularly about our therapy goals and the progress of the child in our sessions. This is especially important when NHS and independent therapists share a case: if communication isn't great, this can lead to therapy which is confusing for both child and parents and may slow down the child's overall progress.

DIFFERENT WAYS OF COMMUNICATING WITH OTHERS

- Face to face: Always ideal, but not always possible, especially for discussing assessment findings, prognosis etc.

- Video calling: The next best thing to face to face.
- Sending videos: Excellent for demonstrating therapy activities to parents.
- Phone calls: Good for discussing assessment results when a two-way conversation is needed.
- Email: Useful for sending longer therapy summaries, reports, and resources, and for forwarding links to useful information videos about SSDs. It is also helpful to follow up after therapy sessions with a written summary of what parents have been asked to do at home, for the sake of clarity.
- Messaging: Often best for communicating about dates and times of sessions, and for late-notice cancellations.

Ensure that at the initial consultation, you discuss and mutually agree the best ways to communicate with the parents/carers and that they know how best to contact you.

PART III

TREATMENT

Chapter 19

GOAL-SETTING

Therapists are used to setting *targets* or *goals*, and we are likely to be familiar with the ideal of goals being SMART – that is, specific, measurable, achievable, realistic, and timely. However, goal-setting is not always straightforward and we can struggle to know where to start when a child seems to have several areas that need working on. We use our clinical decision-making skills to predict whether a goal is achievable or realistic, based on our knowledge of the child and our subjective opinion at the time. We may have to *test out* a goal and then see how the child responds. As therapy progresses and we get to know the child better, our goal-setting skills with the child should improve.

Goal-setting may begin before the assessment period is complete, especially in complex cases, and we may be interspersing therapy with ongoing assessment to gain a more detailed picture of the child. For example, the goal for a preverbal child might be focused on them successfully using an alternative means of communication; however, as they become more verbal, our goals are likely to shift towards more speech-related ones if the child appears to have an SSD.

Goals can be *general* or *specific* and it is usually best to select a small number to start with – perhaps three speech-related goals and possibly up to two others for different areas. Goals can be added, taken away, or amended as necessary, and therapists should not feel that they have to stick slavishly to their original set of goals. Goals should always be shared with parents and teachers, both of whom may also have input into the goal-setting, if appropriate.

Children with special educational needs will have specific individual education plan (IEP) goals which the school will be working on, and SALTs may be asked to contribute towards or help with setting these goals. However, it is unlikely that our therapy goals will be the same as the school's IEP goals, which will probably be more general.

Some published therapy programmes have suggested goal-setting guidance – for example, the Nuffield Dyspraxia Programme (NDP3) and Dynamic Temporal and Tactile Cueing (DTTC). It is suggested that therapists using these programmes read the respective manuals and use the format given.

AREAS WHICH CAN BE INCLUDED IN THERAPY GOALS

- Specific speech production goals: These are the most common ones we think of when working with a child with an SSD – for example:
  - *General* goal: 'X will produce a variety of vowels in CV words.'
  - *Specific* goal: 'X will use "ee" and "oo" vowel sounds, with appropriate lip positioning, following the consonants "m", "t", "b", and "s".'

(Note the use of orthographic spelling rather than phonetic transcription, so that the goals can be more easily understood by others.)

- Intelligibility goals – for example:
  - *General* goal: 'B's connected speech will be intelligible to other children.'
  - *Specific* goal: 'B's connected speech will be understood in 90% of interactions with peers at nursery.'
- Non-segmental areas of speech – for example:
  - *General* goal: 'J will use a variety of intonation patterns in sentences.'

- *Specific* goal: 'J will use falling and rising intonation appropriately to signal statements versus questions with 90% accuracy.'
- Communicative confidence goals – for example:
  - *General* goal: 'V will be a more confident communicator.'
  - *Specific* goal: 'V will read aloud daily in class when asked to do so by his teacher daily.'
- Other areas of language, social interaction, listening skills etc – for example:
  - *General* goal: 'M will make eye contact with the class teacher in school.'
  - *Specific* goal: 'M will maintain appropriate eye contact with the class teacher during carpet time each morning for five minutes.'

Speech goals often target different aspects of speech at different levels simultaneously – for example, single sounds, words, phrases, and conversation – but for different sounds.

HOW THE GOALS WILL BE ADDRESSED

The following decisions must also be made:

- What type of therapy will be used to achieve the goal?
- What games, activities, and resources are needed?
- What cues are needed to support the child in achieving the goal?
- Who will carry out the intervention?
- What carryover work will be needed? Who will carry this out?

Chapter 20

EVIDENCE-BASED PRACTICE

WHAT IS EVIDENCE-BASED PRACTICE?

'Evidence-based practice' (EBP) is a much-used phrase which trips off the tongue and is something that we know is necessary, but can be hard to apply in everyday practice. EBP is a way of using the best external evidence available, alongside the needs and preferences of the client, to make clinical decisions. It involves an awareness of our own biases, a respect for other positions, a willingness to let strong evidence change what is already known, and constant mindfulness of our ethical responsibilities to our clients. If we explore the research evidence, we usually find guidance – although not necessarily consensus – about which therapeutic approach to use. We need to combine an openness to explore and accept new ideas with our own existing therapeutic methods.

EBP is a process and an obligation and should always be used. The onus is on SALTs to apply EBP to each clinical decision made. This is part of our professional responsibility as members of the Health and Care Professions Council (HCPC).

EXAMPLES OF EBP IN SSD DECISION-MAKING

- Which formal assessments should be used for children with an SSD?
- Which areas should be included in the assessment?
- Which questions are relevant when taking a case history?
- How should a differential diagnosis be made?
- How should speech targets be set?
- What therapy method or approach should be used for children with different types of SSDs?

- How frequent should therapy sessions be?
- Is individual or group therapy better?
- Can SALT assistants or teaching assistants be used for therapy?

In certain areas of SSD practice, a considerable amount of research has been conducted into therapeutic methods which are effective or otherwise and we have some clear indicators as to those methods which are likely to work as opposed to those which may not. For example, in the field of CAS and IPD, there has been a lot of research on therapeutic methods and models of delivery – particularly around evidence supporting specific therapy programmes for these subtypes. For other types of SSDs, there are no specific therapy programmes recommended over and above any others, but rather recommendations for the type of *approach* which has been shown to be effective. There are also therapy approaches for which there is *no* evidence base and we should be wary of using these – especially if alternative approaches have a strong evidence base for effectiveness. For many children who may not fit neatly into a single diagnostic group, several therapeutic approaches and models may be available.

DIFFICULTIES WITH LINKING RESEARCH WITH CLINICAL PRACTICE

- Therapists may lack the time to read current research as it is published.
- Some publications are written in non-user-friendly language, which may read as if the intended audience is other researchers, rather than SALTs. This may deter therapists from reading further.
- Some SALTs have not been well trained in how to read scientific papers and lack the confidence to carry out a *critical appraisal* of a paper.
- Many studies focus on statistical detail and lack practical application.

- Research studies often prescribe a high dosage which is rarely possible to deliver in the workplace.
- Children selected for many SSD studies are a homogenous group and may have very similar specific characteristics. In a typical list of referrals, children with SSDs have a much more mixed profile and few would fit the strict research criteria applied in many published papers. We may thus question how relevant some of the research is to a real-life caseload.
- Therapists may lack the time needed to carry out the in-depth assessments recommended in the literature.
- Workload pressures, limited funding, staffing shortages, and waiting lists may be barriers to therapists using EBP consistently.
- Organisations may have a set therapy protocol which prescribes a specific therapy approach or model of delivery, precluding an individual therapist from making decisions based on the individual child – for example, a 'blocks and breaks' model for all children.
- Therapists may feel comfortable with their existing therapeutic practices and lack the confidence to try new techniques.
- 'Tried-and-tested' therapy 'tips' may seem to be effective on their own, without the need to embrace new ideas.

STAYING IN OUR COMFORT ZONE

Most therapists will remember at least some of the therapy methods taught to them during training. The era in which each of us trained will have influenced the types of approaches with which we feel most comfortable, as well as other factors such as the types of clinical placements that we were fortunate enough to experience.

For example, those who trained in the 1980s are likely to have had a much more phonologically based focus, as phonological approaches were at the forefront of research during the 1970s and 1980s. However, this resulted in a bias towards this approach, possibly causing some children with more articulatory SSDs to be (probably unsuccessfully) treated using a contrastive phonological approach. Consequently, many universities promoted phonological interventions and students may not have had as many opportunities to learn about or experience other approaches. Equally, the tendency to follow traditional guidelines may trump the fact that new evidence suggests we should do the opposite. For example, traditional guidelines were to work on sounds that were *early developing, less complex,* and *stimulable in isolation*. However, there is now strong evidence for a different approach which works on sounds that are *later developing, more complex,* and *non-stimulable*.

Straying outside our comfort zone is something about which we should be intentional: we should not only hold onto the therapy style and approach to which we are accustomed but also continue learning and attempting other approaches. Familiarity with an approach is fine, provided that we keep exploring new ideas as they are developed.

For example, my training and clinical placements did not involve any tactile involvement with the child's face/mouth, and I had to build confidence and a new mindset to be able to adopt a new style of therapy which included tactile cuing.

HOW TO MAKE EBP HAPPEN

EBP is a necessity, not an optional extra, so here are some suggested ways of making it more workable:

- Read the RCSLT position papers on SSDs and CAS: These are written by leading experts in the field, are underpinned by a considerable amount of research evidence, and are excellent overviews of current advice and recommendations.
- Participate in or start up a journal club for other SALTs interested in SSDs: Each month, a therapist can read and present a paper on SSDs and discuss it with the group to explore practical, identifiable goals to implement in therapy, including how to adapt the therapy approach to an individual situation and cultural setting.

- Participate in a continuing professional development (CPD) group to share new therapy approaches and to evaluate the evidence in favour of and against their use.
- Join and attend one of the local or national Clinical Excellence Network groups.
- Attend a course on a totally new and different therapy method for SSDs and share what you learn with your colleagues or local group.
- Critically examine how you make clinical decisions and practice, explaining to others the reasons for those decisions.
- Refer to 'What works', a research report by Law et al (see the references at the end of this section), which identifies 57 interventions and explores the level of evidence supporting their effectiveness.

Some of these methods may already be in place within many organisations; however, many therapists working independently, or in small teams with limited time to meet, will need to be more intentional when planning how to make EBP a reality. Keeping updated with new research and ensuring that therapy is evidence based does not necessarily mean reading the original research papers in their entirety, although it is highly recommended that therapists do sometimes read the full paper.

REFERENCES

Law et al (2012). 'What works': Interventions for children and young people with speech, language, and communication needs. Department for Education Research Report DFE-RR247-BCRP10a.

Nuffield Centre Dyspraxia Programme Ltd. NDP3 (Nuffield Dyspraxia Programme Speech Assessment). www.ndp3.org

RCSLT (2024). New speech sound disorders guidance published. www.rcslt.org/news/new-speech-sound-disorders-guidance-published/

RCSLT (2024). Position paper on Childhood Apraxia of Speech (CAS). www.rcslt.org/wp-content/uploads/2024/02/RCSLT-Childhood-Apraxia-of-Speech-CAS-Position-Paper-2024.pdf

Chapter 21

CHOOSING AN INTERVENTION

WHERE TO START

To date, over 40 different intervention approaches have been identified for children with SSDs and the number continues to grow. However, despite the evidence that many interventions are effective, no single approach has proven to be the *most* effective. It may feel overwhelming trying to decide how to approach a child's speech difficulties when several areas are affected or in very complex cases. Clinical decision-making involves choosing from among the available alternatives and collecting, interpreting, and evaluating data to make an evidence-based decision.

When deciding on the best intervention to use with a particular child, it is helpful to look at the following areas and use these in combination to make our decision.

INTERVENTION CHARACTERISTICS

- Whether the specific intervention focuses more on early speech development (eg, first words), the 'phonemic' period (when children are establishing their phonemic system in words and simple phrases), or the 'stabilisation' period (when children are generalising to more complex structures or situations).
- Which stage or stages of production the intervention targets – planning, programming, or execution.
- Which outcome or outcomes the approach targets – speech perception, speech production, phonological awareness, other spoken language skills, or literacy.

Following assessment, analysis, and diagnosis of the child's speech patterns, the choice of intervention will be narrowed down to a smaller group of possible approaches that are suitable. From among this group of possible interventions, we can look at those with the strongest evidence for use with a child whose characteristics align with those for which the approach was designed. We thus need to look at the child's characteristics to continue the decision-making process.

CHILD CHARACTERISTICS

- The child's phonological system and characteristics of their SSD (eg, diagnosis, severity, and the particular speech profile they present with).
- The child's age, maturity, attention, eye contact, and ability to engage with structured speech activities.
- The child's co-occurring difficulties (eg, dyslexia, ASD, listening and attention difficulties).
- Cultural and linguistic factors, and the home environment.
- Parental preferences and ability to carry out follow-up work in between sessions. This also includes available support from school and other support workers (eg, assistants) as an integral part of the intervention.
- The child's preferences – their preferred activities and play style.
- The child's communication needs overall, in terms of current priorities.

As children with SSDs are not a homogenous population, these factors are highly relevant when deciding on the best intervention.

CLINICIAN CHARACTERISTICS

- Knowledge and understanding of the intervention, both theoretical and practical.
- Training received and practical experience in how to carry out the intervention with fidelity.

- The confidence of the clinician in carrying out the intervention effectively.

Interventions with a high level of efficacy in the research can be replicated only if the therapist follows the method with fidelity, which includes correct procedure, dosage etc. Therapists have a responsibility to learn new therapy interventions thoroughly before attempting to use them with a child. This may involve attending training courses or masterclasses, reading the manual, and practising on peers. This will help to build up skills and confidence, and the therapy is thus more likely to be effective.

AVAILABLE RESOURCES

- The time available to carry out the intervention with the necessary frequency and length of sessions.
- The staff available to carry out the intervention with fidelity – these may include SALTs, teaching assistants, parents, or SALT assistants.
- The necessary equipment and materials needed for the intervention – for example, an iPad or other hi-tech equipment.
- The available finances (either within the organisation funding the therapy or the parents themselves).

Although these resource issues are not within our control, they are a necessary consideration, as we need to be realistic and not embark on an intervention if we don't know whether the necessary resources will be available.

COMBINING CHARACTERISTICS TO MAKE A DECISION

These four areas should be considered together to identify the intervention which is the best fit for the child. We need to go through this careful clinical decision-making process for each child and the decision is not static, but should be constantly reviewed and may change depending on the stage of therapy that the child is in. A different intervention approach may be needed at different points of the child's therapeutic journey or as their primary needs change.

It is not acceptable or ethical to use therapy programmes in a prescriptive way to fit specific groups of children – for example, by using minimal pair intervention for all children with phonological delay or the NDP3 for all children with CAS.

DOES IT WORK?

As a wide range of evidence-based approaches have been documented, we shouldn't find it difficult to select a method or approach which is designed for the type of SSD that we are working with. If the therapy that we have chosen seems to be working, that's great and we should stick with it. However, if it doesn't seem to be working, we may need to change our approach, which may mean re-examining our diagnosis and being prepared to re-evaluate our thinking. It is not advisable to use a therapy approach which is not evidence based, and we should challenge the use of such programmes or techniques in the profession. However, if a new intervention has been developed but there is not yet a strong evidence base, one option is to *trial* it and monitor the outcomes carefully.

We should be able to explain to others *why* we are using intervention X and not intervention Y. Going through this evaluation process ourselves and being able to explain and justify our decisions to others helps us to become more skilled and analytical decision-makers.

WHEN A PARENT REQUESTS A SPECIFIC THERAPY APPROACH

There may be times when a parent approaches us, having read up about a specific therapy programme or approach, to request that we use it with their child. If the approach is in line with our clinical decision-making after assessing the child, that's fine; but if not, we have a professional duty of care to explain why this is inappropriate. There may be times when we need to explain that the wrong approach could cause the child 'harm', as we would be neglecting our duty of care to them. Each child deserves the very best therapy from us, without compromise.

Chapter 22

THE CENTRAL ROLE OF PARENTS/CARERS

THE IMPACT OF SSDS ON PARENTS

Anyone who has worked with children who have difficulties in communicating will have experienced the impact that this can have on parents. Anxiety levels may run high – especially at the beginning, when a parent knows that something is wrong but doesn't yet know how it will affect their child long term or whether they will ever become verbal communicators. We can never overestimate the impact on parents of severe SSDs in particular. Parents may experience the full range of reactions, ranging from fear, anger and distress to denial, frustration, guilt, and blame. They may be desperate to find out *why* their child has an SSD and worry that it is their fault. They may blame their partner, or their parents may blame them. Family dynamics can get very complex when emotions are fraught. In other situations, we may have very little contact with the parents if we are working primarily in schools, and it can be hard to feel connected to the whole family and for them to be fully part of the therapeutic process. In some cases, parents may be unconcerned and genuinely feel that there isn't a problem – especially if they have always been able to understand their child.

THE THERAPIST/PARENT PARTNERSHIP

The relationship with parents begins from the moment the parent refers their child or from the first contact in a clinic-based assessment. It is vital that we build a positive relationship of trust so that the parent understands that we know what we are doing, and that there are always things we can do to help and support them, and to work with the child's speech. Parents usually need reassurance right from the beginning that we have the skills and the knowledge to do what we are doing. This is why we have a professional obligation to ensure that we are suitably qualified and experienced to work with each child and their family. If we realise that we are lacking the necessary knowledge, skills, or experience, it is our responsibility to pass on the case to another therapist. This is particularly important in complex cases which may need specialist skills, such as cleft palate, feeding, augmentative and alternative communication (AAC), or CAS.

This relationship of trust is needed so that parents can fully buy into the therapeutic process; and if they trust us, they are more likely to carry out follow-up work according to our instructions. Parents need to feel that the process involves us, the child, and them, so that it can work well and be most effective.

WHAT WE CAN DO FOR PARENTS

- Reassure them that their child will make progress (even if this is not to a 100% level).
- Give them practical ideas on what they can do at home to support their child.
- Help them to realise that their role is valuable and essential.
- Help to reduce feelings of guilt.
- Provide a safe space in which they can express their feelings about their child's communication difficulties without fear of judgement.
- Provide equipment, resources, and games.
- Provide theoretical background, where necessary, as evidence to support the choice of therapy.
- Answer their questions honestly and with confidence.

WHAT PARENTS CAN DO FOR US

- Turn up for sessions.
- Adapt their communicative style towards their child in accordance with our advice, if necessary.
- Carry out specific follow-up work at home with their child.
- Keep records of progress.
- Report back accurately on progress in between sessions.
- Communicate with school/nursery and pass on relevant information from us and to us.
- Keep us informed of any changes in health status, hearing test results etc.
- Always maintain a positive attitude towards their child and their speech.

OTHER FAMILY MEMBERS

Other significant family members, friends, or carers may also be involved in the therapeutic process. These include grandparents, aunts/uncles, childminders, nannies, and au pairs. Our therapeutic relationship with the main person/people who bring the child to therapy sessions is the most important one. It can be difficult to maintain good communication with several people who bring the child at different times, but the child's progress is likely to be better if we can work hard on this.

WAYS OF COMMUNICATING WITH PARENTS/CARERS

If face-to-face communication is not always possible, a quick email or message after each session with a summary of what we have done and what the follow-up work is will be invaluable. Even if the parent has been at the session in person, they may have been overwhelmed with information or struggle to remember everything, so again, a quick reminder of the session in an email can help with this. For school-based therapy, it is helpful to send a brief email summary to the school and parents. It is so quick and easy now to download and send an e-resource to parents; and if an activity is quick and easy to practise at home, it is more likely to be done. Very clear instructions are needed about exactly how to carry out an activity: we have probably all fallen into the trap of sending home a pack of pictures on the assumption that the parent would know what to do with them, only to find that the parent did nothing because they didn't know how to carry out the activity.

Chapter 23

PRE-VERBAL INTERVENTIONS

SSD OR NOT?

One feature of SSDs is that children are very often late talkers; however, when a child is pre-verbal, we don't know whether they have an SSD or whether it is an expressive language delay in the absence of a co-existing SSD. Parents will need a clear explanation of why we cannot yet diagnose their child with any specific speech or language disorder, other than describing what is obvious – that is, delayed expressive language. Over time, the picture will become clearer; and when the child begins to use spoken language, we will hear whether their speech sounds are affected or not.

WHY A CHILD MAY BE PRE-VERBAL

There are many reasons why a child is not talking at an age when this would be expected, including the following:

- Global developmental delay.
- Hearing loss.
- Autism.
- Selective mutism.
- Expressive language delay (with no obvious cause).
- Expressive language disorder.
- Environmental deprivation.
- Other environmental factors (eg, lack of opportunity to communicate).
- Structural abnormality on the vocal tract.
- Neurological disorder.
- Severe SSDs, including CAS.

DOI: 10.4324/9781003480778-27

However, there may already be some early signs, or 'red flags', which may alert us to an increased risk of an SSD.

RISK FACTORS FOR SSDS IN A PRE-VERBAL CHILD

- A history of feeding problems (eg, sucking, chewing, choking).
- No babbling or very little babbling noted by parents.
- Limited vocal play in terms of quantity and variety of sounds used.
- Intent to communicate but lack of imitation.
- Visible 'groping' when trying to imitate sounds or words.
- Significant family history of SSDs.

THERAPY INTERVENTION FOR A PRE-VERBAL CHILD

ENSURE THAT THE CHILD HAS A REASON AND AN OPPORTUNITY TO COMMUNICATE

Working with the parents is essential to ensure that they are increasing the opportunities for their child to communicate – for example, leaving gaps in the conversation for the child to add a sound or word. The SALT may demonstrate different games and activities which might allow space for the child to respond – for example, filling in an animal sound or word at the end of a phrase, or when sharing a picture book. Some parent/child interaction therapy is particularly useful when working with pre-verbal children.

INTRODUCE AN ALTERNATIVE MEANS OF COMMUNICATION EARLY ON

This is essential to prevent or reduce frustration in both the child and the parents, as well as to increase the likelihood of the child having a go at talking. It may be necessary to work with the parents to help them understand how important it is to encourage *any* form of successful communication in the child, rather than just focusing on *spoken* language. Other means include symbols, gesture, signing, and pointing. Parents are often anxious for their child to use speech; if so, it is important that they don't put pressure on the child to speak and, in the process, deter the child from having a go. The benefits of encouraging all forms of communication should be discussed with parents/carers and nursery staff, if appropriate.

If there are signs that the child has a severe SSD, such as severe CAS, and is struggling to produce intelligible speech, a speech-generated device may be considered. This may also be the case if a child has a severe SSD associated with a known neurological impairment. This is a specialist area for SALTs and the child will need a specialist AAC evaluation to determine which device would suit them best. The factors which will be considered include the child's motor skills, the presence or otherwise of any other sensory deficits, the portability of the system, the ease of learning how to use it, and the availability of communicative partners. Speech-generated devices may be 'mid-tech' systems, such as simple apps with voice output which allow a child to put a series of picture symbols together to form sentences, with new vocabulary added as needed. However, it can be difficult for children to understand these systems and locate symbols quickly, and a high level of teaching time may be required. 'High-tech' systems or apps are highly flexible and can be programmed to a child's individual needs, can help with language development, and may interface with other technology. However, they are expensive, and considerable time and expertise are needed for them to be used effectively.

AAC may be used temporarily, to give the child an opportunity to communicate before their speech and language develops further; or permanently, where a child may have persistent difficulties with verbal communication.

WORKING ON LISTENING AND ATTENTION

If this is highlighted as an area of difficulty for the child, listening and attention games and activities can be demonstrated to parents and others, and discussions can be had around promoting a culture of listening, waiting, and not interrupting. Many children with SSDs have difficulties in this area and it will be beneficial for the child in future to have well-developed listening and attention skills. It is also a prerequisite for children to have sufficiently well-developed listening and attention before they can engage with more formal structured therapy sessions.

LANGUAGE DEVELOPMENT

If a pre-verbal child appears to have age-appropriate receptive language, the SALT can begin work on developing some first words in collaboration with parents. This area is usually very much within most therapists' comfort zone, so details are not discussed here. If the child appears to have other areas of communication difficulty, such as a delay with receptive language or social communication, or if they have other developmental differences, these should become the primary focus of intervention.

EARLY SOUND-MAKING

Playing with sound is an important part of early speech development in young children. Babbling is particularly important for practising phonation, articulation, and respiration in a rhythmic style. Children should thus be given the opportunity to experiment with sound as often as possible in play situations. This should include not only practising syllable sequences but also experimenting with different volumes, pitches, intonation patterns, and length of vowels.

Here are some ideas for early sound-making:

- Encouraging repetition of environmental sounds: Taps dripping, car or train sounds etc.
- Volume, pitch, and vowel length experimentation: Using different voices for different characters in books or when watching TV programmes; using long/short 's' sounds to represent long and short snakes.

- Intonation variation: Encouraging imitation of 'oh' using different intonation patterns, using a visual representation such as a mountain, slide, or ladder picture to represent up/down intonation.
- Babble play: Parents can be encouraged to use simple babble sequences themselves and to repeat back any babble sequences that their child attempts.

RHYME AND SYLLABLE AWARENESS

These areas can be introduced to very young children in a play context. Awareness of syllable boundaries is an important skill which is helpful for developing speech beyond CV level. It is also important for spelling when children are older, particularly for words of two or more syllables. Early work on syllable awareness can start with banging a drum or clapping, with the adult drawing the child's attention to the beats. Beating out rhythms for songs and rhymes also provides a rhythmic 'frame' for word and syllable production.

Rhyming is likewise a valuable skill – particularly for helping children to make sense of spelling rules in English and to spot common spelling patterns in words. Rhyming can be introduced early on by teaching children nursery rhymes and reading books which are based around rhyming.

A NOTE ABOUT NON-VERBAL ORAL EXERCISES

To date, there is no evidence that working on non-verbal oral movements is effective in addressing SSDs. Nonetheless, exercises such as sucking, blowing, and tongue movements are still sometimes used by therapists with children who have SSDs in the belief that this might help to increase articulator 'strength' and 'coordination'. However, speech does not require increased 'strength' from articulators; and even if it did, such exercises would not bring about increased strength. Even if a muscle required 'strengthening', we would need to carry out very frequent repetitions of the movement against resistance. Unfortunately, the myth surrounding the value of such exercises persists and it is not uncommon for parents to report that nurseries have been carrying out oromotor movements in the belief that this will help a child's speech production. We know that practising some of the tiny movements required for speech will *not* automatically generalise into speech, which is a highly integrated task. The way in which the nervous system organises *non-speech* versus *speech* movements is very different.

A few exceptions exist, however, as follows:

- Oromotor exercises may be a way to start off a session with some fun movements to help the child 'warm up' and focus on what will be happening in the session.
- In one specific therapy programme, DTTC, one way of preparing the child for saying a particular word is to mouth it before adding voicing. This can help the child in transitioning from no movement at all to speech.
- Oromotor movements form an important part of speech assessment, especially when looking for evidence of oral dyspraxia. The difference between 'assessment' and 'treatment' should be explained to parents, as they may assume that oromotor tasks they have observed in an assessment session are something that they should practise at home.

Generally, however, non-speech oral exercises should be avoided; and this should be explained to parents and nurseries also, so that valuable time is not wasted on unhelpful interventions.

Chapter 24

PHONOLOGICAL APPROACHES: INTERVENTIONS WITH A STRONG EVIDENCE BASE

There are many different interventions devised for children with phonological impairments – too many to describe here. However, a few are discussed in this section and therapists are encouraged to read further/attend courses about other interventions which are evidence based.

CONVENTIONAL MINIMAL PAIRS INTERVENTION

One of the oldest, best-known, and most widely used approaches for phonological intervention, this helps the child to learn the phonological system of their language/languages. A 'minimal pair' is a pair of words that differ by a single phoneme, so that the difference is enough to signal a change in meaning. The words produced as homonyms by the child are paired in rhyming contrasts – for example, 'saw' and 'door' may both be produced as 'door', so this pair of words can be presented to the child, who then learns the phonemic contrast between them. The pairs of words may differ either by one phoneme (with one or more feature differences) or by the presence or absence of a phoneme. In this approach, the pairs of words used are all meaningful words. The use of word pairs produced as homonyms by the child forms the basis of *teaching moments* – that is, moments when a verbal or non-verbal pragmatic cue is given to the child which requests clarification. Examples include: 'Did you mean tea or key?' (verbal cue) or a confused facial expression (non-verbal cue). At this point, the child may be able to self-correct and change their output to produce the correct word. The key point here is that the child makes the link between the fact that their *output* affects the *meaning*, and that producing the incorrect word in the pair causes the listener to misunderstand. The child learns that by correcting their original production, they can communicate the right message to the listener.

The idea is that by working with a small set of minimal pair words, there will be generalisation within that class of sounds and, depending on which stimuli are chosen, across classes as well.

This approach is used for children who have consistent phonological processes or pattern-based errors, which may be either common delayed phonological processes or more unusual processes. It is effective for children with a wide range of severities of phonological impairment; however, there is some evidence that if a child has a severe phonological impairment involving large collapses of contrast, they may benefit more from a different type of intervention to start with – for example, the multiple oppositions approach – moving onto the conventional minimal pairs approach once they have made some progress. It is also not suitable for use with children who have significant motor speech difficulties. Children should either be stimulable for the target phonemes or show evidence of being able to imitate or use cues to produce the phonemes. If a child cannot produce the target phoneme at all, it is unclear as to whether the primary difficulty is phonological or articulatory. However, there is also a version of the minimal pairs approach, called the *perception-production* version, which includes work on fostering stimulability and the more articulatory aspects of producing the contrast.

There are also other types of minimal pair sets of words which form the basis of two non-homonymous approaches to intervention, which are discussed later in this section.

The method for this approach is as follows:

- Choose the target word pairs and prepare appropriate pictures. If there is only one process operating, this is more straightforward – for example, if the child is fronting all velar to alveolar sounds, we can use pairs such as 'tar'/'car', 'tea'/'key' etc. Different phoneme pairs which are affected by this process can be used together – for example, t/k, d/g, n/ng – although with this approach we should not mix up minimal pairs for different processes. If the child has several phonological processes operating, we can either choose the one which would be earlier in the developmental sequence or choose a later-developing process to work on first (using the *complexity* approach rationale); current research has shown that the latter approach may be optimal. It is also better to prioritise non-developmental over developmental error patterns.

- Familiarise the child with the words which relate to the pictures and do a 'listen and pick-up' activity, which ensures that the child knows the names of the pictures and can perceive the difference between the words.
- If the child is not readily stimulable for the target sounds, further 'listen and pick-up' tasks can be done, as perception training can facilitate stimulability. Then try cueing the child to help with accurate production of the words (like articulation therapy at a single-word level), gradually reducing the cueing until the child can produce the words spontaneously.
- Use different games and activities in which the child has to produce the correct target word when both pictures are presented (eg, through posting games, sorting, fishing, lotto games) and use cueing where necessary – for example: 'Did you say pin or bin?' 'Is it the quiet sound or the loud one?'
- Generalisation beyond the single-word level can be achieved through games and activities that involve phrase and sentence production.

This intervention should be carried out primarily by a SALT, although parents and schools may be able to do carryover work with some explanation and training. Children who progress with the first phonological process can then move on to the next one. It may take weeks or months to establish each contrast, depending on factors such as the frequency of therapy, the age of the child, and the amount of appropriate carryover work in between sessions.

MULTIPLE OPPOSITIONS INTERVENTION

This is a contrastive phonological intervention for children with moderate to severe phonological impairment and there is a growing evidence base for this approach. It is designed for children who have collapses of contrast due to many phonological processes operating simultaneously. This may be consonant substitution, deletion, or both. For example, a child who is stopping all fricatives and fronting all velars, and who has final consonant deletion, and context-sensitive voicing, would say 'dough' to mean 'toe', 'dough', 'go', coat', 'cope', 'goat', 'so', 'foe', 'show', and 'soap', among many other words. In this case, many adult phonemes are produced as a single sound, which causes a high level of contrast loss, leading to significant unintelligibility.

In multiple opposition intervention, which is a variation of minimal pairs intervention, multiple sounds from across the child's phoneme collapse are targeted simultaneously. This has been found to be a highly effective intervention for facilitating systemwide change in children with phonological impairment. It is based on the idea that phonemes are contrastive to signal differences in meaning; and that selection of targets that are maximally distinct from each other, and from the child's errored production, means that the targets are more salient to the child and can thus be more easily learned.

Up to four target sounds are chosen from one rule set and five sets of minimal pair words are created, which contain the child's targets and their current realisations of those targets.

For example, if a child has a very limited phonetic inventory and uses 'd' in place of all velars, affricates, and clusters, the target sounds chosen could be 'g', 'st', and 'j', so a set of target words to use might be:

- Dough – go, stow, Joe.
- Do – goo, stew, due.
- Deer - gear, steer, jeer.
- Door – gore, store, jaw.
- Day – gay, stay, jay.

The method resembles the conventional minimal pairs approach described earlier, although additional support may be needed in the form of imitation and simultaneous production with the therapist.

COMPLEXITY APPROACH

The goal of this approach is to improve intelligibility by promoting systemwide gains in a child's sound system. The theoretical basis is that by focusing on more *complex* targets rather than *simpler* ones, we do not have to work on the less complex structures; these will naturally develop as the more complex structures are achieved. The evidence for this approach is strong. It goes against the traditional approach, which advocates that we should start with *simple* targets and work towards more *complex* ones.

Complexity can refer to phonetic complexity, phonemic complexity, or syllabic complexity.

At the phonetic level, targets chosen are often ones which are not present in the child's phonetic inventory and which are consistently in error, non-stimulable, and late acquired. This contrasts with the more traditional developmental approach, which favours sounds that are inconsistently in error and stimulable, and that usually develop at an earlier age. At the phonemic level, targets are chosen which belong to more complex, later acquired groups of sounds – for example, affricates rather than fricatives (as the learning of affricates should also promote the learning of fricatives). There should be maximal voice, place, and manner feature differences, and the target sound need not be paired with the child's substitute sound. At syllabic level, complex clusters can be used, rather than singletons or less complex clusters. Also, non-words can be used in this approach.

Treatment includes imitation, moving onto spontaneous training, and targets starting at word level, rather than at single-sound or syllable level.

CYCLES APPROACH

This is a phonological remediation model designed for children with highly unintelligible speech (severe to profound expressive phonological impairment); it is also used for children with special aetiologies. The goal is to enhance and promote the accuracy and consistency of speech sounds and patterns within a cognitive linguistic framework.

The targets are carefully selected earlier and later-developing sounds. Phonological patterns are identified which are stimulable and are presented in a cyclical way. The phonological patterns are then recycled as needed in subsequent cycles, with the inclusion of more complex but achievable patterns and levels (eg, clusters and liquids) at the right moment.

There is evidence of the effectiveness of this approach in individual and group treatment – including for children with other impairments, such as cleft palate – and progress is significantly better with stimulable sounds.

METALINGUISTIC APPROACHES

This involves the therapist and child talking and thinking about the properties of phonemes (place, voice, and manner), the structure of syllables, and communicative effectiveness. The focus is on the child understanding how these properties of speech effect *meaning* through a system of contrasts. The child can then actively revise and repair their own error productions to produce accurate words and thus meaning.

Many other interventions have been reported; this section has merely introduced a few which are more commonly used. Therapists are encouraged to read further and explore other techniques.

USEFUL RESOURCES

Bowen, C (2015). *Children's Speech Sound Disorders* (2nd ed). Wiley-Blackwell.

Bowen, C. Speech-language therapy dot com. https://speech-language-therapy.com. This website has an extensive set of resources, including many pictures which are free to download and print.

Williams, AL, McLeod, S, and McCauley, R (eds). *Interventions for Speech Sound Disorders in Children* (2nd ed). Paul H. Brookes Publishing Co.

Chapter 25

PHONOLOGIAL APPROACHES: SYLLABLE-LEVEL INTERVENTION

This approach focuses on phonotactic structures – that is, structures at the syllable level. This includes patterns such as:

- Initial consonant deletion.
- Final consonant deletion.
- Reduplication.
- Weak syllable deletion.
- Monosyllables only.
- Cluster reduction.

Some ideas for working on these areas are presented below; they can also be addressed using some of the interventions in Section 24.

INITIAL CONSONANT DELETION

- Reinforce any initial consonants in CV syllables, regardless of accuracy.
- Start with consonants already in the child's inventory.
- Increase the child's awareness of the presence or absence of initial sounds in syllables.
- Model pairs of words with an initial sound versus an open syllable (eg, 'bee'/'ee', 'moo'/'oo'), and talk about how they look and sound, using language such as: 'Look at my lips close for m'; 'Can you hear there's a "b" sound here … ("bee"), but not here … ("ee")?'
- Use sequences of words which have a CV, V, CV, V pattern for the child to imitate (eg, 'bee, ee, bee, ee, bee, ee').

- Facilitate production of CV patterns by starting with VC combinations in strings (eg, 'um-um-um-um' can be repeated and gradually shaped into 'mum-mum-mum-mum' and then into 'mum').

FINAL CONSONANT DELETION

- Reward *any* final consonant, even if it is not the correct one.
- Talk about the 'last' or 'end' sound in the word (older children may find it helpful to see the word written down as an additional visual cue for learning the difference), and allow the child to hear lots of examples of 'sound at the end' versus '*no* sound at the end' (eg, 'baa'/'bark', 'car'/'calm').
- Focus on sounds already in the child's inventory and start with the most common ones in the child's language (in English, these are fricatives, velars, and voiceless plosives).
- Use syllables with *short* vowels first (eg, 'miss', 'hot', 'bap', 'bike').
- Move on to long vowels and diphthongs when the child can use some final consonants with short vowels.
- Practise sequences of CV-CVC-CV-CVC words (eg, 'bye, bike, bye, bike').

REDUPLICATION

- This occurs when the first syllable in a two-syllable word is repeated – for example, 'daddy' is produced as 'dada', 'water' becomes 'wa-wa' etc.
- We can take advantage of the tendency that young children have to use /i/ as the second vowel in two-syllable words (so 'horse' may become 'horsie' and 'duck' may become 'duckie'). If we choose words that naturally have /i/ as the second syllable, but have a different first syllable, children may find it easier to produce these two-syllable words accurately. If we also use an alveolar as the consonant in the second syllable, followed by /i/ (as these sounds often co-occur in English), we are creating a facilitative

environment. Early target words could thus include 'busy', 'messy', 'body', and 'bunny'.

WEAK SYLLABLE DELETION

- Children often only delete weak syllables if the stress pattern of the word is *weak-strong* (eg, 'be**cause**', 'gi**raffe**', 'pre**tend**'), rather than *strong-weak* (eg, '**bis**cuit', '**or**ange', '**fizz**y'). This is known as an *iambic* word. We can help the child to produce these words in phrases by making the whole phrase iambic, which may help the child to use the correct stress pattern to keep the rhythm going. An example phrase might be: 'I **cry** be**cause** I'm **sad**', or 'I **saw** a **big** gi**raffe**'.
- Clapping out and saying the word simultaneously is another commonly used technique and miming a clapping motion can be used as a visual cue for a child who needs prompting to remember the weak syllable.

MONOSYLLABIC WORDS ONLY

- When children use only monosyllabic words, they can be encouraged to develop two-syllable words by using target words that are often duplicated by children anyway (eg, 'poo-poo', 'wee-wee', 'bye-bye', 'choo-choo'). These can then be changed by one consonant or vowel so that the syllables are different.

CLUSTER REDUCTION

- The evidence is in favour of us initially choosing clusters to work on which are more *marked*, to facilitate generalisation; three-element clusters may be better to work on before two-element ones.
- S-clusters are not considered as 'true' clusters and working on these is less likely to facilitate system-wide change. However, they are often easier for children to produce, as they are more visual and can be a good introduction to the concept of a 'two-step sound'.

USEFUL RESOURCES

Bowen, C. Speech-language therapy dot com. https://speech-language-therapy.com. This website has a wide selection of free-available resources and pictures for SSD work.

Chapter 26

INTERVENTION FOR INCONSISTENT PHONOLOGICAL DISORDER

A QUICK REMINDER ABOUT IPD

IPD is due to a deficit in the phonological plan, or template, which results in a combination of error types with variability of production of single words which is equal to or greater than 40%. This can be measured using the DEAP assessment. There are also likely to be other error types present, such as typical phonological processes or more unusual ones. Care should be taken to ensure that the differential diagnosis is correct, especially as *inconsistency* is present in the speech of other children with SSDs who do not have IPD.

IPD affects intelligibility significantly, as the inconsistency means that it can be very difficult for other – even familiar – adults to tune into the child's speech due to the lack of predictable, consistent patterns.

ONE EVIDENCE-BASED APPROACH

Only one evidence-based therapy approach has been shown to be effective with IPD: CVI. A significant body of research has shown that this approach is effective both for IPD and for inconsistency of speech production with other groups of children. It is not, however, recommended for use with CAS; although in the very early stages of therapy, when children with CAS have a very limited vocabulary, it has been found to be a useful tool. It is also not effective with children with other types of SSDs, such as articulation disorder or CPD.

The reason why such a specific intervention is recommended is because the impairment in IPD is an impairment in *phonological planning* (ie, an impaired ability to plan the sequence of phonemes that make up a word), which results in inconsistent productions of the same word. CVI is recommended by the RCSLT as the evidence-based intervention to use for IPD. Children with IPD are resistant to phonological contrast or articulation therapy.

CORE VOCABULARY INTERVENTION

WHEN TO USE IT

CVI can be used in three main scenarios:

- Where IPD had been diagnosed in a child from age three, following assessment that has shown inconsistent errors at a frequency of 40% or more.
- Where IPD is suspected but the therapist is unsure. It may be that the IPD/CAS distinction is unclear.
- Where a child has CAS but has a very limited vocabulary. In this case, CVI may initially be used to establish a small set of intelligible words. However, it is not effective as an ongoing therapeutic approach for CAS.

The child should also be able to engage with some level of structured therapy that involves word repetition and imitation. This approach is suitable for a wide range of ages and cognitive abilities. It is also important to evaluate the contextual factors (personal and environmental) before deciding whether this is an appropriate intervention – partly because it involves a high level of daily home practice and is a family-centred intervention. The child should also have adequate hearing levels: however, it has been successfully used with children who have an identified hearing impairment.

HOW IT WORKS

The aim is to develop consistent production of whole words, rather than accuracy of individual sounds. As the speech of children with IPD cannot be analysed using error patterns, the approach uses single words which are not necessarily related to each other and are treated as individual units to be worked on. The focus is on establishing consistency using individualised, high-frequency, highly functional, powerful words. It targets the underlying impairment, which leads to improved intelligibility. This intervention helps the child to assemble a specific sequence of phonemes for a particular word that can be used consistently in different utterance contexts. The number of words worked on is limited and they are drilled until consistently used accurately, although developmental errors may be acceptable. The focus is on targeting *consistency* of production over and above 100% articulatory accuracy, as consistency significantly affects intelligibility. Studies have found that consistency generalises to other untreated words. Generalisation of consistency is expected once the child can produce at least 50 words consistently.

DOSAGE

The recommendation is for individual, twice-weekly sessions lasting about 30 minutes each. Significant progress should occur within 16 half-hour sessions, which should be sufficient to attain consistent production for both the target words and generalisation to untreated words. Progress will vary according to the practice in between sessions, the age of the child, the severity of the SSD, and other factors related to motivation.

TARGET SELECTION

After assessment and diagnosis, but before the first therapy session, the child, family, and teacher are asked to select a bank of 70 high-frequency functional words for the child. These should be words that have the most immediate and relevant impact on the child's ability to communicate and participate – for example, the names of key people in the child's life; favourite foods, toys, and places; and function words/phrases such as 'please', 'thank you', and 'sorry'. If possible, the words should contain a range of different sounds, syllable shapes, and syllable numbers. The use of functionally powerful words is motivating for both the child and the family, as consistent production of these types of words increases functional communication. These will be the main stimuli words used in the intervention sessions. Careful explanations are given of the importance of aiming for consistency, but that the child's production may not be error-free.

WEEK 1, SESSION 1

In the first session, about ten target words are selected randomly from a set of 70 target words. The bank of 70 words is chosen by the child, parents, and teachers to be the focus of intervention.

The therapist teaches the child to produce each of the ten words using the very best consistent production possible, through feedback and cueing. This may include the use of verbal prompts, visual cueing, tactile cuing, letter-sound correspondence, talking about syllable number or phoneme number in the word, placement, manner, voicing, and length cues. Other techniques, such as backward chaining, may also be used. Each word may be taught 'sound by sound', taking each syllable at a time. It is important to help the child to build their own phonological plan, rather than just giving them the phonological plan to start with and asking them to repeat the whole word. This may include feedback such as: 'You used "d" instead of "s" – let's try it with "s" at the beginning instead.' Once the *best production* of the word is established, multiple repetitions of the ten words are elicited and practised in games for the rest of the session. The parent and/or teacher then practises the ten words with the child every day until the next session, focusing on establishing *consistency* of production and encouraging the child to produce the very best production they can each time. For example, if the child has been able to produce the word 'bus' accurately in the therapy session, the parent/teacher should ensure that the child says it this way every time at home; if they deviate from this, they should be given feedback and cueing to help them produce it accurately.

If the child is unable to produce a particular target word accurately in the therapy session, perhaps due to an additional articulatory difficulty, the therapist will allow the child to use their *best version*, which is the version that parents and teachers should subsequently aim for in between sessions. If the child can improve on their original version, this new production then becomes their *best version* and the aim is for the child to produce this new realisation of the word consistently. Lots of positive feedback during sessions is important.

WEEK 1, SESSION 2

In the second session, the therapist tests the child on the ten words from the previous session. Each word is tested three times, with the trials separated by another activity. The newly learned words are drilled and practised in games with opportunities for lots of repetition, and feedback is given about consistency if the *best production* is not produced. The aim is to elicit over 100 repetitions per session. The words should also be elicited not only in single-word naming activities, but also at phrase and sentence level when single words are consistent. The intervention may need to be adjusted depending on how the child and family are progressing.

WEEK 2, SESSION 1

The child is asked to repeat the stimulus words from the previous week three times and words which are now produced consistently are removed from the list. Words produced inconsistently return to the bank of words and can be worked on again in subsequent weeks. The above format is repeated each week, introducing a new set of ten words each week for the first session; for session 2, the same format is repeated as for week 1, session 2.

MONITORING PROGRESS

CVI is designed to last approximately eight weeks, with two sessions each week and a vocabulary bank of 70 words. Every four sessions, a set of ten untreated words should be elicited three times each to monitor system change and thus generalisation. When the production of untreated words becomes consistent, the DEAP inconsistency subtest can be carried out, which should confirm that generalisation is occurring.

When consistency is established, the child may have some remaining speech errors which are more consistent, such as common developmentally delayed patterns. These can be worked on separately using different techniques such as phonological contrastive therapy, perhaps a few weeks after the CVI has been completed.

TROUBLESHOOTING

The success of this intervention depends primarily on the initial diagnosis of IPD being correct. If the child does have IPD and the therapy is carried out according to the guidelines, there should be rapid progress within the timescale given. If there is not, this may be due to one or more of the following reasons:

- The child may have been incorrectly diagnosed with IPD and may have another subtype of SSD which requires a different therapy approach (eg, CAS).
- The family/teacher may have been unable to carry out the necessary practice in between sessions.
- There may be behavioural, motivational, or developmental reasons as to why the child is not making the expected progress.
- The dosage that the therapist can provide or the number of sessions that the family can attend is not adequate to allow sufficient progress in therapy.

In these cases, every effort should be taken to ensure that the above reasons are explored – especially if there is doubt over the accuracy of the original diagnosis, which may have to be re-examined.

It may be possible to use CVI successfully with a variation of the above guidance – for example, if only one session per week is possible. There is some evidence of the effectiveness of this approach using a similar but not identical programme of intervention.

It should also be noted that progress has been observed across the languages of multilingual children, as this intervention does not target the language-specific phonological system, but rather phonological planning ability, which crosses all languages of an individual child.

CASE EXAMPLE

Jake was late saying his first words and when he started to use a small vocabulary of words, they were unintelligible, even to his parents – a cause of frustration for both Jake and his family. He was first referred to speech and language therapy by his mother at age two, as he was very quiet, and advice was given on facilitating early language development. He was reviewed at 2.6 years and assessed using the TPT, which showed a high level of unusual sound substitutions and lots of inconsistency. It was hard to make a differential diagnosis between CAS and IPD, as Jake was reluctant to imitate words or have a go at spontaneous naming; however, the SALT decided to start some CVI therapy, beginning with a small set of high-frequency, functional words chosen by his mother. He responded quickly to this therapy and within six weeks, he had developed a set of 20 intelligible words which were produced consistently. After three months of twice-weekly therapy, Jake had made significant progress with both expressive language and intelligibility and no longer met the criteria for a diagnosis of IPD. He did have some delayed phonological processes, which were worked on at age four, and he responded well to therapy. By 4.6 years, he was age appropriate with his speech sound development and was discharged.

USEFUL RESOURCES

Online courses are available via Course Beetle which provide more detailed training on how to use CVI. See www.coursebeetle.co.uk for details.

Chapter 27

THERAPY FOR ARTICULATION DISORDER: PRINCIPLES

WHAT IS ARTICULATION DISORDER?

Articulation disorder is the inability to produce a perceptually acceptable version of a particular phoneme, either in isolation or in any phonetic context. Accurately distinguishing phonological from articulatory errors is crucial before we start therapy, as the treatment approaches are very different. If the child can produce a particular phoneme in isolation and in two or more vocalic positions, the speech error is phonological rather than articulatory.

OVERVIEW OF INTERVENTION APPROACH

- A primarily *motor-based* approach is needed.
- Auditory perception of speech sounds may be a secondary focus.
- Therapy is usually structured, with repetition and drills needed.
- The intervention approach is based on behaviourist principles and operant conditioning, especially to establish accurate production of a sound in isolation.
- Principles of motor learning are often applied for generalisation and maintenance.
- The approach is eclectic, having been around for many years.

BEHAVIOURIST APPROACH (FOR LEARNING A NEW SOUND)

This is effective for achieving accurate production of a phoneme in isolation. It involves giving cues to the child about how to position their articulators, starting with imitation, and then providing feedback each time they attempt the sound, including details about success or what to change. The feedback is frequent, immediate, and focused on their 'performance' – for example: 'That was good – you pushed your lips out.' Practice usually follows a 'blocked' schedule (eg, 20 repetitions of the same sound), targets are simple to begin with, and practice is constant.

MOTOR LEARNING (FOR GENERALISATION AND SELF-MONITORING)

Feedback is infrequent (not after every attempt by the child) and delayed (by a few seconds). Feedback focuses on *knowledge of results* rather than *knowledge of performance*. The practice schedule is random rather than blocked, and this approach uses variable practice and complex targets.

EXAMPLE OF USING A BEHAVIOURIST APPROACH FOR PRODUCTION OF /k/

Goal: To produce /k/ so that the child can replace the previously incorrect sound (/t/) in every position of the word, in every sound combination, and in every speech situation.

- Perception (auditory discrimination):
    - Identify, name, and discriminate the sound in error form from other sounds in increasingly complex contexts. For example, present /t/ and /k/ as single sounds for the child to point to the correct letter or picture representation of the sound. Repeat this with CVs, VCs, and CVCs. Start with identification of the correct sound in the therapist's production and then in the child's own production.

- Production: This involves a series of consecutive constructive steps. The child is required to analyse, compare, and vary the phoneme until accurate production is achieved.

Steps: Production of /k/:

- In isolation.
- In VC position (eg, 'ark', 'eek').
- In CV initial position (eg, 'car', 'key', 'core').
- In VCV position (eg, 'akar', 'eekee').
- In longer words, clusters, and different positions (eg, 'camel', 'baker', 'caterpillar', 'cloud').
- In two-word phrases (eg, 'two cars', 'blue key').
- In longer phrases and sentences (eg, 'The baker's cat is driving the car and eating a carrot').
- Generalised to different conversational and situational contexts, and with time pressure.

PRINCIPLES OF MOTOR LEARNING IN ARTICULATION THERAPY

This approach is becoming very popular in the field of articulation therapy and is the basis of several published programmes for CAS. The principles of motor learning can be applied to learning any new motor skill, such as learning to produce a speech sound consistently in conversation. The initial stages of learning to produce the sound in isolation to begin with are best carried out using a more behaviourist approach; but once the child can produce the sound and needs to learn how to generalise it, this approach is highly effective.

The principles of motor learning focus on the type, frequency, and timing of *feedback* given to the child, and the type of *practice* carried out. This approach has a strong evidence base.

FEEDBACK

This refers to the way in which we respond to the child's attempts at achieving the target. It is usually verbal, but may be tactile, gestural, or visual.

- Learning has been found to be more effective when feedback is *infrequent*. Feedback should not be given every time a child says the target word, but rather after every few attempts.
- Feedback should also be *delayed*, but this should be gradually introduced. The delay should be a few seconds.
- The child should be given *knowledge of results* through comments such as, 'That sounded really good' (as opposed to comments on *performance*, such as, 'Good job – you really pushed your lips forwards then').

PRACTICE

This refers to the way in which a child practises their target in sessions:

- *Random* practice is when the child practises a target just once, rather than in blocks of ten or 20, randomly throughout the session. The target may be practised lots of times during the session, but with other targets in between. At this stage, the child should be getting more consistent with their production, as opposed to when they are still learning to say a target word accurately.
- *Variable* practice involves changing aspects of the target other than the sounds themselves – for example, by practising it with different volumes, pitches, intonation patterns etc. This helps the child to acquire and use different motor programmes and means that the target can be generalised more effectively.
- When a child is learning a sound or word initially, we usually start with simple targets that gradually become more *complex*; however, when we have reached the generalisation stage, the targets should be more complex for learning to be effective and generalisation to occur, as we need to mimic the complexities of conversational speech as much as possible.

> In articulation therapy, it is key that there are *multiple accurate productions* of the target as, according to motor learning theory, it is through frequent repetition of the correct version that the child is able to learn and generalise this production into spontaneous speech.

SUMMARY OF ARTICULATION THERAPY PRINCIPLES

As we move the child through the different stages of therapy for a particular area of articulation work, we shift gradually from using behaviourist principles to motor learning principles, as summarised in Table 27.1.

OTHER THERAPY APPROACHES

- Ultrasound biofeedback supporting articulation therapy: This is a highly effective method and may provide greater generalisation than articulation therapy alone; however, most children and therapists have limited access to this technology.

Table 27.1 Summary of stages of articulation therapy principles

Beginning of therapy (eg, learning a new sound) Behaviourist principles	Later in therapy (for generalisation) Principles of motor learning theory
Feedback: - Frequent - Immediate - Knowledge of performance	Feedback: - Infrequent - Delayed - Knowledge of results
Practice: - Blocked schedule - Constant practice - Simple targets	Practice: - Random schedule - Variable practice - Complex targets

- Myofunctional therapy: This approach is popular with some therapists and requires additional training and experience to carry out. There is currently insufficient evidence that myofunctional therapy directly enhances treatment outcomes for articulation disorders.
- Prompts for Restructuring Oral Muscular Phonetic Targets (PROMPT): This is another approach requiring additional training. While there is insufficient evidence about its effectiveness, it is popular with some therapists who report a high level of effectiveness with certain children.
- TalkTools: This method is used by a small number of therapists and includes the use of small instruments which are designed to help the child achieve accurate articulatory placement for sounds. Again, there is insufficient evidence to support the use of this technique.
- AI-based automated therapy tools: In the last few years, there has been an increase in research into the development and use of AI in SSD therapy, particularly with articulation disorders. This has come about primarily through advancements in automatic speech recognition (ASR). Many researchers have proposed AI-based tools – fully automated systems available through mobile-based or computer-based applications – which can detect subtle differences in the speech production of children and give feedback, so that the child can practise without the need of adult intervention. Some success has been reported, although we are still a long way off from these tools gaining widespread use in clinical practice. As yet, there has been insufficient research comparing AI-based automated therapy and direct therapy from SALTs, and it is unlikely that there will ever be a time when AI 'takes over' the role of SALTs.

Chapter 28

THERAPY FOR ARTICULATION DISORDER: COMMON SOUND ERRORS

These are some practical ideas for eliciting 's', 'r', 'sh', and 'k'. One important point is that the sound should be *perceptually acceptable*, rather than being produced with a specific articulatory position and movement. There is considerable variation between people as to how they produce a sound.

General principles for eliciting speech sounds include the following:

- Use verbal phonetic placement cues – for example, describing the lip and tongue positions, manner, and place of articulation.
- Use visual cues such as gestures, picture representations of single sounds, and requests for the child to watch your face carefully.
- Use successive approximation and shaping from sounds which the child can already say.
- Use 'facilitating contexts' – for example, using back vowels to elicit velars and front vowels to elicit alveolars.

Eliciting 's'

- Lengthen 't' by saying it slowly and gradually lengthening the friction (eg, ts, tss, tsss).
- Shape from 'ts' (eg, 'cats').

- Model a 'lazy s' or 'sleepy s'.
- Lift the tongue up so that the sides touch the back teeth and the tip is behind the top front teeth (also try with it behind the lower front teeth), and pull back slightly, close the teeth a little and then blow air slowly towards a centrally placed finger.
- Smile when saying 's' and then add a close front vowel afterwards (eg, 'sea').
- Encourage the child to close their teeth together in cases of interdental substitution. This should be phased out as soon as possible, however, to prevent incorrect jaw position being established.
- For lateral 's', use a short straw held on the top teeth so that air can be directed through the straw to make a whistle. This helps the child to redirect the airflow centrally rather than laterally.
- The 'butterfly procedure' may be used for lateral 's' (see the references at the end of this section).
- Try with the tongue first behind the top teeth and then behind the bottom teeth (as for some children, it is more natural for it be behind their bottom teeth).

Eliciting 'r'

- Touch the alveolar ridge with the tongue, then curl back and away.
- Make a 'growly' sound (eg, a roaring lion or a dog growling).
- Start with tr, dr, shr, cr, or gr, as this can help with better placement.
- Use a 'smiley' mouth (as opposed to lip rounding for 'w'); however, be aware that this lip position in CVs works only when the following vowel is a high front vowel /i/.

- Shape from 'ah' (lift the tongue up and then lift the tongue sides to touch the molars).
- Shape from 'l' (say a long 'l' and then drag the tongue tip slowly back along the roof of the mouth until it drops to 'er', then shape from 'er' to 'r').
- Shape from 'er' (lift the tongue and pull back).

Eliciting 'sh'

- Shape from 's' – move the tongue back slowly along the roof of mouth and round the lips.
- Elicit 's' and then add 'y' to follow the 's'. If these sounds are then sequenced quickly, especially in the medial position, an approximation of 'sh' can be achieved which can then be shaped.
- If the child can produce 'ch', the second element of this sound can be prolonged.

Eliciting 'k'

- Start with an open back vowel, 'ah', and then add 'k' ('ark').
- Use 'r' blends to give a velar nature to the 'r' (eg, 'crow', 'cry').
- Use gravity to help allow the tongue to fall naturally into a back position by modelling a 'tipped back' head position.
- Encourage the child (or parent) to push their finger or thumb down onto the front third of the tongue and then try saying 'k'.
- Touch the neck under the jaw near the throat to feel movement.

- Shape from velar nasal.
- Produce 't' with the tongue behind the lower incisors and lift the back of the tongue.
- Cough or gargle.

FACTORS AFFECTING GENERALISATION

It is sometimes quick for a child to learn a new sound and begin combining it with a vowel to make simple syllable shapes. At this point, it is tempting for both therapists and parents to breathe a sigh of relief that the child has mastered their new sound. However, it is usually at this point that the hard work begins, as the generalisation of the sound into harder words and phrases, and then fully into conversation in all contexts, can be a long process.

Factors affecting this include the motivation of the child and parents, the consistency of home/school practice, the frequency of therapy sessions, and the number of accurate productions of the target elicited during each session. Some children find it particularly difficult to generalise their 'new' sound into conversation and it may take many months, or even years, for it to be generalised.

CASE EXAMPLE

Nosheen was referred at age ten by her mother as she was unable to produce 'sh', either in isolation or in any word position. This was causing her significant anxiety and affecting her confidence with speaking in front of groups of children at school. Assessment showed that her difficulties were only with articulation of 'sh' and she could produce 'ch', 's', and 'j' appropriately. During the initial assessment session, the SALT used 'ch', which she was able to make, and encouraged Nosheen to say it as a 'lazy ch' so that it sounded like 'sh'. She managed this very successfully and said her name accurately for the first time ever. She then had one further session during which she practised tongue twisters and reading aloud, which showed that she was able to use 'sh' at sentence level but needed occasional reminders in conversation. Her confidence levels had increased significantly in just ten days, and her mother was given advice on helpful verbal cues and asked to contact the therapist if there were further concerns in the future.

Chapter 29

TREATMENT APPROACHES FOR CAS

CAS has already been described in Section 7 as a rare, high-need, and complex speech disorder, which can be difficult to diagnose accurately. As the impact on a child with severe CAS is significant, there has been a lot of research into effective therapy approaches to treat children with CAS. There is a general consensus that no one therapeutic method of treatment for CAS is accepted as the ideal or recommended method, but the published efficacy studies to date support five well-documented therapy approaches or programmes which are effective – all of which are recommended in the RCSLT position paper on CAS published in 2024.

Apart from these five specific methods, there are also other treatment principles and techniques which have been identified in the literature for children with CAS or phonological disorder, and for when these overlap. A small number of children do present with a 'pure CAS' profile and for these children, one of the five well-documented programmes is recommended. Most children who present with CAS symptoms also have a unique combination of difficulties with articulation, phonology, and phonological awareness, so these children may benefit from therapy – which is well established in the literature – using some of the principles described in earlier sections of this book.

NUFFIELD DYSPRAXIA PROGRAMME

The NDP3 was developed in the UK by Pam Williams and is well known and widely used around the world. It provides a set of therapy procedures and techniques to plan and implement treatment for children with CAS, from single-sound production to sentence-level and connected speech. Picture resources are provided to use in therapy sessions and for home/school practice. A detailed assessment is also included which facilitates the setting of goals and the monitoring of progress.

The NDP3 is most suitable for children aged three to seven, although it has been shown to be effective with children up to age 12. Children should be able to sit and concentrate for at least short periods of time, and to engage in structured speech work and accept feedback from the therapist. They should also be able to manage picture-based presentation and have, or have the potential to develop, some 'meta-linguistic' skills, such as understanding about blending and segmenting speech sounds, syllables, and words. The NDP3 can be used not only with children who have CAS, but also with those who have other types of SSDs.

The following principles underpin the NDP3:

- It employs principles of motor learning: It is primarily a *motor* intervention and the terminology and concepts come from the principles of motor learning. This a well-established theory which describes how a new motor skill can be learned using a hierarchy of pre-practice and practice phases, with carefully planned specific cues and feedback given to the child on their performance and results. Tasks are broken down into finely graded, achievable steps and each therapy session aims at a high number of repetitions.
- It uses psycholinguistic principles: The aim is to build accurate motor programmes, using a high level of repetition, practice, feedback, and cueing.
- A bottom-up approach: The NDP3 uses the concepts of building a 'brick wall', with single sounds at the bottom; then CV syllables and single words; then more complex phonotactic structures; and finally, phrases, sentences, and connected speech at the 'top' of the wall. Higher-level skills are seen as being dependent on the lower levels being learned. Therapy aims to 'fill the gaps' in the wall.
- A multi-level, multi-target approach: Treatment planning involves using assessment findings to identify the starting

point for a child. Four stages in treatment planning are proposed and target areas are set at one or more areas of the hierarchy. Children may be working at different target areas at different levels – for example, a single sound in isolation plus a voicing contrast at CVC level.

There are four stages of treatment, as follows:

- Stage 1: Establishing a core set of single sounds, CV syllables, and CV words, and introducing some basic intonation work through working on pitch, volume, and vowel length. Single sounds are represented by picture symbols and there are worksheets for sequencing single sounds to make CVs and then practising CV sequences.
- Stage 2: Building CVCV and CVC structures.
- Stages 3 and 4: Producing multisyllabic words, clusters, phrases, and sentences, with suggestions for generalisation into conversation.

Therapists are recommended to attend an NDP3 training course and purchase the manual with assessment and therapy materials.

DYNAMIC TEMPORAL AND TACTILE CUEING

The DTTC method also uses the principles of motor learning theory and was designed and developed by Edythe Strand in the US. It is aimed at young children with severe CAS, who are either non-verbal or have very limited verbal output, and who have significant difficulties with imitation. It has also been found to be effective for children who have responded very slowly to other types of therapy and remain highly unintelligible. Older children with less severe CAS presentation may benefit from a different therapy approach.

The key components of this approach are as follows:

- It focuses on *movement, not sounds* – movement transitions are worked on primarily.

- It aims to improve motor planning.
- It uses a variety of cues to aid accuracy of movement, including tactile, gestural, and auditory cues.
- It is a face-to-face therapy style, which requires direct eye contact from the child to maximise visual cues.
- Therapy goals and the choice of target words/phrases and cueing used are based on the outcome of *dynamic assessment*.
- It requires a very intensive therapy schedule, with four sessions of direct therapy per week recommended, all of which must be carried out by SALTs rather than parents or other professionals.

Dynamic assessment, in this context, is the process of testing out the cues which help the child to improve their production of a target word, rather than them naming a picture unaided. This process is key to choosing stimulus words for therapy and knowing which cues to use in sessions.

Initial stimuli are carefully chosen which are functional, use a variety of vowel shapes and phonotactic structures, and combine easier and trickier consonants and vowels. A small number of stimuli are selected and as therapy progresses, further words are added, with an ongoing focus on practising these stimuli using different volumes and intonation patterns.

The steps involved in the actual therapy process are very specific and each should be followed for each stimulus word/phrase chosen as follows:

- Imitation.
- Simultaneous production with prolonged vowels – this can be done if the child cannot imitate. The therapist and child say the word simultaneously at a slower rate, with the addition of tactile and/or gestural cues as necessary. The child should maintain correct jaw and lip postures, even when the rate is slowed.
- Reduction of vowel length – vowel length becomes gradually shorter, but still with simultaneous production.

- Rate is gradually increased to normal rate, with simultaneous production maintained.
- The therapist reduces the volume of their loudness, eventually to miming, to facilitate independent production by the child. The therapist finally mouths silently, but with continued cues given.
- Direct imitation – the child imitates immediately after watching the therapist saying the word first. If the production is incorrect, the therapist may move back several steps and repeat. Varied intonation and volume are also practised.
- Introduction of a one or two-second delay – the therapist ensures that the child waits for one or two seconds before imitating.
- Spontaneous production – single words or phrases are elicited spontaneously by encouraging the child to finish off the line of a phrase, song etc (known as a *cloze* task).

DTTC is becoming more widely used in the UK as more therapists become trained in this approach. Training videos are available, as are a small number of masterclasses for therapists who want to develop their skills further. DTTC is a therapy tool which has a solid theoretical basis and a strong evidence base; however, the number and frequency of sessions required are high, which may be difficult for many therapists to implement in practice.

RAPID SYLLABLE TRANSITION TREATMENT

Rapid Syllable Transition Treatment (ReST) was developed in Australia for CAS and focuses on prosodic and segmental aspects of speech. It was designed for school-aged children and is more suitable for older children or those with milder CAS.

Its key features are as follows:

- It uses the principles of motor learning.
- Complex, varied, multisyllabic non-word strings are practised intensively.

- Non-words are used to avoid interference from the lexical or semantic system, or ingrained error patterns on familiar words.
- Random sequences of syllables are practised, allowing lots of new motor plans to be laid down.
- There is generalisation to real word production and connected speech.
- High-level, one-to-one input from a SALT is needed and home practice is not given.

The steps involved in this approach are as follows:

- A series of CVCVCV nonsense words is practised, in which all vowels and consonants should be different (eg, 'tapoonee', 'codarnoo', 'feleedow'). If the child is struggling to produce these accurately, CVCV words should be practised initially.
- When accuracy has reached 80%, the complexity of the word is increased – for example, by adding a consonant cluster or by putting the stimulus word in a carrier phrase (eg, 'spincroobar').

The child's production of each word is considered 'accurate' when the three consensus CAS characteristics identified by ASHA are managed simultaneously:

- Articulation: This refers to the accuracy of the segmental aspects of the word (referred to as 'sounds' with the child).
- Lexical stress: The child must mark the strong syllable and use the schwa correctly in weak syllables. Increasing the pitch, loudness, or duration of stressed syllables, relative to unstressed ones, will achieve lexical stress accuracy (syllables are referred to as 'beats' with the child).
- Syllable transition: Syllable transition accuracy is determined by a smooth, normal-rate production of the word with no hesitations, restarts, or staccato speech (syllable transition is referred to as 'smoothness' with the child).

These three aspects of the child's speech production are discussed with the child when feedback is given, and the terms 'sounds', 'beats', and 'smoothness' are used to clarify which aspect of the word needs correcting.

The ReST website contains videos, a step-by-step description of how to implement ReST, a 'readiness' checklist to use with a child, a parent handout, and a clinician self-assessment. The information and videos on the website are sufficient for SALTs to be able to begin using this approach with children who have CAS without further training.

INTEGRATED PHONOLOGICAL AWARENESS

Integrated Phonological Awareness (IPA) is a linguistic intervention programme, devised in New Zealand, for pre-school and young school-aged children with speech and language impairment. It has been found to be effective when used with children diagnosed with CAS, and improvement was found with speech production as well as early reading and spelling development. It is more suitable for children with less severe CAS and/or older children. IPA is not underpinned by motor learning theory, so it is distinctly different from the previous three approaches. This approach is not widely used in the UK, compared with the NDP3, DTTC and ReST; but it is included here as it is one of the five evidence-based interventions for CAS, as mentioned in the RCSLT position paper on CAS.

ULTRASOUND BIOFEEDBACK

This is the final and most recent evidence-based technique for treating CAS. Ultrasound shows real-time articulatory movements, and a visual display provides specific information about the articulatory parameters required to produce accurate speech. The technology converts high-frequency soundwaves to images and the contour of the tongue can be displayed, showing important information about tongue shape during speech. Motor learning principles can be applied to this approach. The evidence base for this approach is growing and is mainly based on single case studies.

Although this method is highly effective, its use is limited by the cost and location of the equipment, which is not usually available in most local clinics and schools, or for therapists in independent practice. However, it may be possible for children to access this technology in larger practices or national specialist centres.

OTHER PUBLISHED THERAPY PROGRAMMES

There are several other published programmes which are designed for children with CAS and other SSDs; however, there is limited evidence of their effectiveness for CAS. They may have some value for other groups of children with SSDs or children who have a mixed profile of speech impairments with elements of phonological and articulatory involvement.

Examples of these include the following:

- Melodic intonation therapy uses melody, rhythm, and stress to improve functional speech production.
- PROMPT is a tactile method based on touch, pressure, and kinaesthetic and proprioceptive cues.
- The Cycles approach is a linguistic approach targeting phonological error patterns for children who have poor intelligibility and several error patterns in their speech, including CAS.

Courses are available on PROMPT and the Cycles approach for SALTs who want to explore these further. However, as there is limited evidence of their effectiveness, there should be particularly good reasons for choosing either of these approaches and parents should be made aware of the research evidence and the reasons for the use of the approach with their child.

Case example

Daniel was diagnosed with CAS at age seven. The Covid-19 pandemic meant that face-to-face therapy had to be postponed and he started receiving teletherapy during this time. Previously, Daniel had received a variety of different therapy approaches; however, when his CAS diagnosis was confirmed, he started working with a new therapist who introduced a structured NDP3 approach. This was highly effective, although he had some residual articulatory distortions which required some additional articulation work. At age eight, Daniel had acquired all segmental aspects of speech, although his intelligibility was still variable at times. He continued some further work monthly to focus on awareness of rate and use of pauses. This work was primarily carried out through reading aloud. He also had some therapy on production of polysyllabic words and phrases, using the 'everyday phrases' and 'complex sentences' sections of the NDP3, as well as some work on tongue-twisters and poems. Daniel continued to have monthly teletherapy sessions to review progress and provide further strategies to help him be more intelligible in conversation.

USEFUL RESOURCES

Murrell, K (2024). *Working with Childhood Apraxia of Speech*. Routledge.

REFERENCES

Apraxia Kids. Dynamic Temporal and Tactile Cueing (DTTC): A treatment approach for severe CAS. https://www.apraxia-kids.org/webinar_library/dynamic-temporal-and-tactile-cueing-dttc/

Gillon, G and McNeill, B (2007). Integrated Phonological Awareness: An intervention program for preschool children with speech-language impairment. University of Canterbury, New Zealand. www.canterbury.ac.nz/content/dam/uoc-main-site/documents/pdfs/d-other/01-Integrated-Phonological-Awareness-Manual-Sept-07.pdf

McCabe, P, Thomas, D, Murray, E, Crocco, L and Madill, C (2017). Rapid Syllable Transition Treatment – ReST. University of Sydney. https://rest.sydney.edu.au

Nuffield Centre Dyspraxia Programme Ltd. NDP3 (Nuffield Dyspraxia Programme Speech Assessment). www.ndp3.org

Queen Margaret University (2015). Ultrasound Visual Biofeedback Treatment for Speech Sound Disorders in Children. https://www.hra.nhs.uk/planning-and-improving-research/application-summaries/research-summaries/ultrasound-visual-biofeedback-for-speech-sound-disorders-in-children/

RCSLT (2024). Position paper on Childhood Apraxia of Speech (CAS). www.rcslt.org/wp-content/uploads/2024/02/RCSLT-Childhood-Apraxia-of-Speech-CAS-Position-Paper-2024.pdf

Chapter 30

PHONOLOGICAL AWARENESS INTERVENTION

PRINCIPLES OF DEVELOPING PHONOLOGICAL AWARENESS SKILLS

If a child has been assessed as having difficulties with phonological awareness – especially if they have a phonological component to their speech disorder and/or literacy difficulties – the following activities can be worked on, depending on the child's age and level of difficulty. It is necessary to have completed an initial phonological awareness assessment, so that activities can be targeted at the appropriate level. These activities can also be carried out alongside production work.

These activities are fundamentally *auditory*, although it can be helpful to use some visual cues to aid understanding of the tasks – for example, by using counters to represent syllables or showing them the front and back of a car to demonstrate initial and final sounds.

The sequence of these activities is based on the stages given in the Newcastle Intervention for Phonological Awareness and involves the use of 'scaffolding' to support the child in learning each step, such as saying the words together or modelling the required response.

- Syllable awareness:
  - This can begin with awareness of the number of words in a simple sentence and build up to identification of syllable number in two, three, and four-syllable words.
  - Initial syllable deletion: This is the ability to listen to a word, delete the initial syllable, and say the remaining

portion of the word accurately. It should start with simple two-syllable compound words and then move on to non-compound words – for example: 'Can you say "cupcake"? Now say it again, but don't say "cup".'
- Final syllable deletion: As above, for final syllables.
- Initial and final syllable deletion in words of three or more syllables.
- Phoneme identification:
  - Identify the initial sound in CV and CVC words, starting with a choice of two phonemes and then increasing the number of options.
  - Identify the final sound in VC and CVC words, as above.
- Phoneme deletion:
  - The child has to say the word without the initial sound – for example, 'What's the first sound in "bake"? Now miss out the first sound and it makes …?' Start with real words and move on to non-words.
  - The child says the word themselves and deletes the initial sound.
  - As above, for word-final sounds.
- Phoneme substitution:
  - Swapping one sound for another, starting with initial sounds – for example: 'Say "dog" – now miss off the "d" and say "f" instead.'
  - As above, for final sounds.
- Rhyme identification:
  - Identifying whether two words rhyme when the adult says the words.
  - Identifying which two words rhyme from a list of three (said by the adult).
  - As above, but using pictures, and then from their own production of the words.
- Consonant cluster identification and manipulation:
  - Naming both sounds in a two-consonant cluster.
  - Deleting the first and then the second sound in a cluster and saying the new word.

- Substituting one phoneme for another in a consonant cluster and saying the new word – for example: 'Can you say "green"? Now take away the "g" and say "p" instead' (preen).

USEFUL RESOURCES

Newcastle Phonological Awareness. About the NIPA. https://research.ncl.ac.uk/phonologicalawareness/assessmentandintervention/aboutthenipa/

Chapter 31

WORKING WITH OLDER CHILDREN WITH SSDS

WHY WE MIGHT WORK WITH OLDER CHILDREN

Older children (ie, age seven and upwards) may have ongoing speech sound difficulties due to an ongoing disorder which was identified at a younger age or may not have been referred until later. Late referrals often happen because the child's speech difficulties were not of concern when they were younger, as parents may have felt that the child would 'grow out of them', or because they were mild enough not to have been noticed at a young age. Other reasons include lack of access to a SALT service earlier on, or issues with other areas of communication (eg, language delay) that were more noticeable and thus 'masked' an underlying SSD. Schools sometimes observe difficulties with spelling and then identify a difficulty with production of a specific sound, resulting in them querying the child's phonological awareness and articulation of that sound.

AREAS COMMONLY WORKED ON WITH OLDER CHILDREN

- Articulation of later-developing sounds – 'th', 'r', 'ch', 'j', 's', and 'sh' are commonly worked on at age seven or upwards if they have not yet developed fully by this age.
- Generalisation of sounds worked on at a younger age which have not yet fully generalised at the phrase/sentence level or into conversation.
- More complex sound combinations such as clusters and polysyllabic words.

- Prosody/stress patterns/rate/volume/pitch/voice quality – these are common areas of difficulty in children with CAS but may also affect children with other types of speech difficulties.
- Ongoing phonological delay/disorder – some children may take longer than others to develop a full range of phonological contrasts in their speech.
- Social-emotional aspects of the SSD on the child.

HOW OUR APPROACH DIFFERS WITH OLDER CHILDREN

Therapy with older children is often more structured than with younger children – especially within the school environment, where children are used to concentrating for longer periods of time in the classroom. It is usually possible to elicit more repetitions of the target sound/word/stimulus, and for sessions to be longer and more focused on speech production.

As children get older, they often become more aware of their speech patterns being different from those of other children, which can mean that they find it easier to perceive their own production as being accurate or otherwise and then self-correct. Motivation can be greater and they may respond well to charts and visual displays which show their progress. Once children can read, this extends the types of activities which we can use with them, including reading books aloud, focusing on their target sounds, and word games.

Older children can be more involved in setting goals for therapy, monitoring and reviewing their progress, and taking a more active role in decision-making, such as when therapy should be terminated. Discussion with older children about the emotional aspects of having an SSD is important, and issues such as bullying, coping with teasing, having the confidence to speak in public, and general wellbeing are all important to work on.

IDEAS FOR HIGHER-LEVEL AND GENERALISATION WORK

- 'Silly sentence' games: Use a bag of objects with the target sounds and ask the child to select two or three and make up a sentence using the target words (eg, 'The sausage is sliding down the slide').
- Use a bag of objects to practise saying polysyllabic words. Dinosaurs are popular with some children.
- Tongue-twister books and poems: Children who are fluent readers may enjoy these.
- Topic-specific vocabulary production: Children who struggle with production of longer and more complex words may find it helpful to practise vocabulary specific to their current topics at school (eg, shape vocabulary, mathematical terms, science vocabulary). This makes speech work more functional for them.
- Sections from the NDP3 are useful for children who need to practise complex words at sentence level. The 'everyday phrases' and 'complex sentences' sections are helpful in this regard.
- A bag of objects with consonant clusters can be used to generate sentences with cluster words.
- Fluent readers can read a page of their reading book, paying particular attention to their target sounds. This is useful for carryover work at school, as teaching assistants can combine listening to children read with reminding them about their sound production.

Chapter 32

CONSIDERATIONS FOR CHILDREN FROM CULTURALLY AND LINGUISTICALLY DIVERSE BACKGROUNDS

In many areas of the UK, the SALT caseload has a high proportion of children from culturally and linguistically diverse backgrounds. Children who have more than one ambient language as they are growing up are more likely to present with a different pattern of development in all their languages, as compared with children exposed to only one language.

Guidance from the RCSLT suggests that when working with bilingual children, assessment and intervention should be delivered in both languages. An adequate budget for interpreters, and the additional time needed to liaise with them and provide appropriate assessment, are required to ensure an equitable service. Interventions that facilitate speech development in all languages are likely to have the greatest overall impact. However, this is currently a very tricky situation because the budgets are not available to fund an adequate interpreter service. Discussions are taking place to address this difficulty, but there are no easy solutions, either in the NHS or in the independent sector. The RCSLT advises that our interventions with bilingual children should be 'enabling' and 'normalising', providing solutions where these are available.

SPEECH DIFFERENCES

Knowledge of the local accent and dialect of the area in which the child lives, and the speech patterns in all ambient languages spoken in the child's home, is important when assessing speech, so that any variation due to linguistic diversity is not pathologised as an SSD. Differences may be phonemic or prosodic. One common example is in the London area, where 'th' is often replaced by 'f', and this is often an appropriate substitution which is part of the local dialect. We should never attempt to 'correct' this sound substitution, unless it becomes clear that the child's peers and family members all use 'th', and the child is still using 'f' in place of 'th' over the age of eight.

When children with SSDs speak more than one language, their speech production will be affected across all languages. However, the errors may manifest themselves differently in each language. For example, languages have different ratios of vowels to consonants, and greater or fewer numbers of consonant clusters or polysyllabic words; and there are other differences, such as variations in the types of word structures which commonly occur. Tonal languages will be more difficult for children who have prosodic difficulties. Differences in the speech sound characteristics of languages may thus affect the child's intelligibility in one of their languages more than the other. Children with CAS have been found to favour the language with the easier phonemic inventory and word structure.

CULTURAL DIVERSITY

We should familiarise ourselves with the cultural backgrounds of the children with whom we work and ensure that each child is given an equal opportunity to access SALT services. This includes ensuring that families have access to clear linguistically and culturally appropriate information about our service. All assessment and therapy materials should be culturally appropriate for that child and their family.

USEFUL RESOURCES

HCPC. New standards of proficiency. www.hcpc-uk.org/standards/standards-of-proficiency/

RCSLT. Bilingualism overview. https://www.rcslt.org/speech-and-language-therapy/clinical-information/bilingualism/

Chapter 33

MULTIPLE AREAS OF NEED

Many children referred to us may have SSDs alongside another areas of need, either with related communication needs or otherwise. For each child, we need to carry out a full case history, assess every aspect communication, and be aware of any other areas of development which may impact on our choice or implementation of therapy.

It can be a challenge to identify where to begin when a child has multiple areas of need; but by asking ourselves the question, 'What is the main factor affecting this child's ability to communicate successfully and effectively right now?', we may find the best starting point.

For the purposes of this book, it is not possible to cover all possible combinations of difficulties with which a child may present; however, some of the more common things that are likely to arise in the SSD population are mentioned here.

HEARING IMPAIRMENT

Many children we come across routinely have a history of fluctuating hearing loss due to otitis media and some will have had, or be waiting for, grommets. We do not need specialist training to work with children who currently have, or have had in the past, fluctuating hearing loss. Their difficulties are usually very similar to those of children who have phonological delay or disorder or articulation disorder, alongside language delay, and we can treat them as we would any other child who presents with a delay or disorder.

Children with severe or profound hearing loss need specialist therapy and SALTs require additional training and experience to work with these children. Deafness affects many areas of speech – especially phonological development, articulation development, and suprasegmental aspects of speech. Receptive and expressive language and social interactions are also likely to be affected. Cochlear implants are becoming more common, and work with children who have had a cochlear implant involves a high level of *auditory training*, so that they can possibly learn to detect differences between sounds and words which they were previously unable to detect.

Children with profound hearing loss will also probably need access to signing and sometimes a specialist provision for their education.

CLEFT LIP AND/OR PALATE

Cleft palate may be *syndromic* (associated with a syndrome such as Treacher Collins syndrome) or *non-syndromic* (no known associated syndrome).

A child may already have a cleft palate diagnosis and have had surgery when they are referred to a local SALT service. Cleft palate is a specialist area of work and all cases should be managed by a regional cleft palate team, who are likely to refer on to a local SALT for follow-up work. If this is the case, a report from the specialist SALT in cleft palate, with recommendations, should be available. It is important that the two SALTs involved communicate about the intervention required and work together to deliver the appropriate therapy. There are sometimes post-surgery complications – for example, if the seams have split following surgery, causing a fistula on the alveolar ridge or hard palate. Any signs of this should be referred immediately to the cleft palate team.

It may be that the cleft palate is identified or raised as a possibility by a non-specialist SALT, in which case the child should be referred immediately to the local cleft palate team for a full assessment and diagnosis. Warning signs for the possibility of a sub-mucus cleft include a bifid uvula, or a blue tinge or bump on the hard palate. Cleft lip may be present in isolation or alongside a cleft palate. If it occurs in isolation, it is unlikely to affect speech significantly, especially if timely surgery is successful and the child has full mobility and range of lip movements following surgery.

Cleft palate affects speech in different ways and the following are likely to be impacted:

- Resonance: As the velopharyngeal closure is affected, the child may sound hypo or hypernasal, and there may not be a clear oral/nasal contrast for consonants (eg, 'p' or 'b' versus 'm', and 'd' versus 'n'). This can be assessed by eliciting sentences with lots of 'm' words and then lots of 'p' words. If resonance is affected, there will also be a difference in the quality of a vowel if the nose is held versus not held; this can be assessed by eliciting an 'ee' sound and listening for resonance differences between the child's nose being held or not. Cleft palate is more often associated with hypernasal resonance (ie, too much air is in the nose during speech).
- Nasal emission or turbulence: This may be heard during speech and may or may not be present alongside resonance differences.
- *High-pressure* sounds (eg, 'p', 'b', 't', 'd', k', and 'g') are likely to be more difficult to achieve than *low-pressure* sounds (eg, 'm', n', and '-ng').

Therapy with cleft palate resembles that used for other articulation disorders, so the method usually begins with production of the target sound in isolation and then gradually builds up to different syllable positions and more complex contexts. Cues are used, as appropriate, such as visual, tactile, and auditory cues. Bad habits may form pre-surgery, so the child may need therapy post-surgery to 'undo' some of the poor habits built up as the child needs to learn how to use their new velopharyngeal closure. There may well be 'compensatory misarticulations' which will need therapy to correct. Surgery may not be 100% effective, so the closure may not be perfect straightaway.

A child may have velopharyngeal insufficiency in the absence of a cleft, due to an abnormal structure of the velopharyngeal sphincter, or valve, resulting in decreased speech intelligibility – especially hypernasality, generally muffled speech, and possibly puffs of air, squeaks, or snorts which accompany oral pressure consonants. Velopharyngeal incompetence, in the absence of a cleft, is when there is abnormal movement in the sphincter, resulting in insufficient closure. These types of difficulties can be very difficult to assess and diagnose and require a specialist team with high-tech imaging equipment. It is important to distinguish between nasal emission which accompanies oral pressure consonants and emission which *replaces* consonants, as the management of these is different.

The RCSLT cleft lip and palate guidance has further information on these areas.

AUTISM

Children with autism may have speech difficulties which are known to be related to their autism – for example, prosodic differences, flat intonation, or difficulties with regulating volume. They may also have specific difficulties with regulating their speech to suit the listener and may lack the motivation to change their current speech patterns. Children with autism may also have co-occurring speech difficulties which may present as articulatory or phonological, and we need to decide what the most pressing need is in terms of where to direct our therapy. Our clinical decision-making skills come into play here, and we may decide that working on social communication is the priority. If the child has a significant SSD, however, and has the attention skills and ability to engage with structured therapy, then speech work may be the priority at this time.

DEVELOPMENTAL DELAY

Children with developmental delay may also have speech and language delay or disorder. We may have to adapt therapy activities to suit the developmental level of the child and make allowances for any additional physical limitations or sensory needs. Therapy goals for children with developmental delay or complex needs are likely to include targets which span several different areas of need.

USEFUL RESOURCES

RCSLT. Cleft lip and palate overview. https://www.rcslt.org/speech-and-language-therapy/clinical-information/cleft-lip/

Chapter 34

OUTCOME MEASURES

WHY ARE THESE NEEDED?

Measuring outcomes is a professional requirement of the HCPC, and we need to have data about which interventions work and which don't, so that we know whether our therapy for a particular child is effective or not. This data is also needed for the sake of the profession, to contribute to a fuller understanding of treatment effectiveness. Outcome measures are also important for *reflective practice* (an essential part of our CPD). A vital part of our work is self-evaluation, asking the questions: 'Why was the outcome more or less positive than expected?' and 'What can I do differently?'

PUBLISHED OUTCOME MEASURES

There are many research papers which focus on the therapeutic effectiveness of specific interventions, some of which are discussed in the sections on evidence-based therapy techniques above; however, these measures are often focused on outcomes from very specific therapy programmes which are carried out in a highly structured way. Very little information is available about how we can measure outcomes in clinical practice.

HOW SALTS OFTEN MEASURE OUTCOMES

We are used to target-setting for children, albeit that some therapists use a more structured method of doing this than others. For example, specific targets may be set on a six-weekly or termly basis, with a decision made at the end of this period as to whether the target has been 'met', 'partially met', or 'not met'. This information certainly has some value, in that it shows us, parents, teachers, and others whether the targeted work carried out has been effective. However, this method does not tell us *why* a target has not been met or which *other* areas of communication may potentially have improved as a result of the work we have done on one of the target areas.

PRIMARY OUTCOME MEASURES

These are measures showing the outcomes of specific speech (or other) targets which have been set and worked on during a specific period – for example, 'production of word-final "s" in single words'. These types of measures are most commonly used as outcome measures following a period of therapy and are useful for sharing with others and quoting in reports and progress summaries.

Primary outcome measures include the following:

- Standardised assessments – for example, the DEAP, and comparing the child's standard scores with those of the general population and with the child's previous scores.
- Formal assessments – for example, carrying out a single-word naming assessment and comparing the number of correctly produced words with the previous assessment, or counting the number of correct phonemes and comparing with previous measures.
- Informal assessments – for example, transcribing the child's speech during play or conversation, and comparing speech sound substitutions or speech sound realisations with those prior to therapy.

SECONDARY OUTCOME MEASURES

While these measures are often considered to be of less significance, they are very useful for evaluating how much the intervention is affecting the child's life in other ways. As our aim is to help bring about change in the child's overall communication and quality of life, including their social interactions, these measures are important. It can be tempting to focus on the specifics of the speech goals and thus lose sight of the end goal, which is always successful, meaningful communication. This links in with the WHO's classification system to support health and wellbeing, with reference to the wider impact which a speech impairment has on a child's life.

Secondary outcome measures include:

- Parental rating of intelligibility through rating scales or questionnaires.
- Teacher rating of intelligibility through informal rating in the classroom or questionnaires.
- Intelligibility rating by an unfamiliar listener (eg, by listening to an audio recording of the child or by parents reporting how easily their child is understood by unfamiliar adults).
- Using a social communication rating scale or rating communicative confidence informally or through a rating scale.
- Measuring/counting successful social interactions with peers through classroom or playground observation. This may be done using a specific length of time and a similar context, so that the measures can be repeated at intervals and compared more accurately.
- Psychosocial measures (eg, anxiety rating scales).

USEFUL RESOURCES

RCSLT Online Outcome Tool (ROOT): This supports the collection and collation of therapy outcome measures and the generation of reports which can potentially inform clinical decision-making and demonstrate the effectiveness of different interventions. https://www.rcslt-root.org/Welcome

RCSLT Outcome Measures Checklist: This is helpful in providing different ways of measuring outcomes. https://www.rcslt.org/outcome-measures-checklist/

PART IV

SERVICE DELIVERY AND DECISION-MAKING

Chapter 35

TIMING OF THERAPY

There is a considerable amount of research on the best time to treat different types of SSDs and some very helpful findings can provide us with guidelines for decision-making in this area. There is increasing evidence that by targeting certain types of SSDs at specific ages, we can deliver therapy in the most effective way, using our available resources for the good of the child. It is important that children with SSDs are not treated as if they are one homogenous group in terms of therapy delivery.

EARLY INTERVENTION

This is particularly important where a young child is struggling to communicate their needs, the child is frustrated, and the parents need support and advice on how best to support them. We know the benefits of early intervention in terms of limiting the effects of a communication impairment when a child is older; however, more structured and direct intervention may have to wait until a later stage. Working on articulation of sounds requires a high level of resilience and patience on the part of the child, so delaying therapy until approximately age seven is often recommended. As the presentation of SSDs usually changes over time, different types of interventions may be needed at different points in the child's development.

PRACTICAL CONSIDERATIONS

Factors such as when a child is starting school, changing year group, moving to secondary school, or doing important exams should be considered. There may be a particular reason for focusing on speech in the term before a child starts school, as it would be advantageous for the child to have the chance to catch up with their peers before starting. It may also be more difficult for a child to have therapy sessions outside of school once they are in full-time education. The long school holidays can be a great opportunity to do more intensive work, either on a one-to-one basis or in groups. Other factors affecting the timing of therapy include waiting for a child to have grommets inserted before starting speech sound work, so that they have optimal hearing levels. Therapy may have to be fitted in around other major events in a family's life, such as the birth of a new baby, a house move, or illness in the family. It should be possible to make allowances for these unavoidable events and to be flexible in what we can offer in such cases.

OPTIMAL AGES FOR WORKING ON ARTICULATION OF PARTICULAR SPEECH SOUNDS

There can be expectations from parents, teachers, and others that intervention as early as possible is best for all speech difficulties, regardless of type. Although this is certainly the case for CAS and IPD, the most effective time to work on other areas of speech – such as articulation and certain phonological processes – need not necessarily follow this principle. As time and resources are limited, we must be careful to ensure that our intervention is carried out when it is most likely to be effective, rather than intervening too early, when the child may not be developmentally ready or mature enough to benefit fully. It is also important that we don't intervene at a point when the child is likely to make spontaneous improvements over time themselves – for example, if they are unable to produce a particular sound but are still within the normal range for development of that sound, due to their age.

Articulation of 's' may be affected by *dentition*, so it is often better to wait until the adult teeth have come through before starting to work on this sound. Gaps at the front of the mouth make it much harder for the child to attain and maintain appropriate tongue position. Therapy for interdental lisps and lateral 's' articulation substitution errors is thus more effective from age seven, rather than at pre-school age or in the early school years. Parents may be keen for articulation therapy to take place before age seven, but it is important to explain the rationale for waiting until the child is older, emphasising that if the difficulty is purely with articulation of one specific sound, in the absence of phonological or phonological awareness issues, there is unlikely to be an impact on literacy.

Therapy to work on articulation of other later-developing sounds, such as 'r' and 'th', should also take place from age seven, as the child is unlikely to be developmentally ready before this for the precise movements needed to teach these sounds. Also, if therapy for these sounds is delayed, many children will end up acquiring them naturally before age seven anyway, so therapy may well not be needed at all.

WHEN TO WORK ON PHONOLOGY

There is much more variation in the recommendations for when to work on phonology. Early listening, auditory discrimination, and sound awareness work can take place at pre-school age; and sometimes more direct work on certain phonological processes, such as fronting and stopping, is highly effective at age three or four, depending on the individual child. As phonological delay and consistent phonological disorder may impact on a child's literacy development, earlier intervention at the pre-school level may be beneficial. Even if children are still delayed with their phonology when they start school, it is likely to be beneficial for them to have had some exposure to sound contrasts before they begin their formal education, which places strong emphasis on phonics from the beginning of the reception year. However, children with delayed phonology whose speech patterns do not include non-developmental substitutions respond better to therapy at age five or older, so if resources are limited, it may be a better use of time to wait until these children have reached this age. Many children with delayed phonology at age four make spontaneous progress by age seven and thus do not need any direct therapy intervention.

Children with CPD respond better during the pre-school years, so this cohort of children should be prioritised for direct therapy at a younger age than those with phonological delay. Children with CPD which persists into late childhood have been found to be at greater risk of long-term psychosocial problems, including self-harm, so prioritising these children is important.

IPD is best treated at age three; and as this can often be resolved in a relatively short timescale, it may be possible to discharge these children before they start school.

CAS

As described in the earlier sections on CAS, (see sections 7 and 29), children with this rare disorder need early intervention and should be prioritised for input as soon as possible.

WHEN THERAPY IS NOT APPROPRIATE

There are times when we might assess a child and find that they fall well within the normal range for all areas of communication, including speech sound development. If this is explained to the parents, with the clear message given that if there are any concerns in the future, they can contact the SALT service again, this is usually fine with the parents. Sometimes, however, parents can be highly anxious or overly concerned about what might appear to us to be a very minor, age-appropriate sound substitution or articulation distortion in a young child. We should acknowledge the parents' concern, reassure them, and hand over developmental norms leaflets, if appropriate; but we should not agree to carry out direct therapy with the child. This decision should be the same regardless of whether the parents are accessing therapy through the NHS, a school-based service, or privately. Therapy which is delivered due to parental pressure is not in the best interests of the child and may lead to excessive anxiety in the child.

Chapter 36

DOSAGE

HOW THIS IS CALCULATED

The amount of therapy delivered is fundamental to its effectiveness. Unfortunately, treatment intensity is often driven by service constraints rather than evidence or the child's needs. Intervention is often spread too thinly and fails to have an effect. This leads to children with SSDs sitting on caseloads for far too long, meaning not only that their speech remains disordered for longer, but also that there may be psychosocial consequences for the child. The previous section raised the issue of the *timing* of therapy, which must be addressed initially depending on the type of SSD that is presenting. Once it has been established that the child is at an appropriate age and level of maturity to be able to access direct therapy effectively, we can think about the dosage.

The intensity of therapy can be described in five different ways:

- *Dose*: The number of times you practise an item in a therapy session.
- *Dose form*: The activity that provides the practice.
- *Dose frequency* (or *intensity*): The number of therapy sessions delivered in a specific period of time.
- *Total intervention duration*: The whole time period over which the intervention (or episode of care) is delivered.
- *Cumulative intervention intensity*: Derived from a calculation of *dose* x *dose frequency* x *total intervention duration*, giving us the total number of times that an item is practised over the duration of the therapy.

WHAT DOSAGE IS RECOMMENDED FOR SSDS?

The optimum amount of intervention will vary for each child according to the following factors.

TYPE OF SSD

- Articulation disorder: Variable amounts of therapy frequency and duration are recommended in the literature, from weekly to daily, and from ten-minute sessions up to one hour in duration. The key factor is that there are multiple accurate productions of the target in each session – the minimum number of repetitions recommended is 100. Some studies specify a total number of correct productions needed for a particular sound to be generalised (eg, between 1,900 and 2,300 trials in total).
- CAS: Studies show that frequent therapy sessions are more effective than infrequent sessions. The research evidence for the effectiveness of CAS programmes is based on an intensive level of therapy – for example, four times per week in blocks of 12-15 sessions is optimal for both the NDP3 and ReST. However, a minimum of twice per week is recommended and sessions should ideally be 45-60 minutes in length. Other sources recommend three to five individual sessions per week.
- IPD: For the CVI approach, the recommended dose is twice-weekly therapy sessions of 30 minutes each over a period of 18 weeks.

For other types of SSDs, there are variable amounts of therapy recommended, which are dependent on many other factors.

RESPONSE TO INTERVENTION

Often, our therapy decisions are based on how a child responds to the intervention. It is rarely possible to predict at the assessment stage how many sessions a child will need. It is often only once therapy is underway and we can see how the child is responding in terms of motivation, engagement with the therapy sessions, and speed of progress that it becomes clear how much therapy will be needed. This is one reason why it is so hard to plan the number of therapy sessions in advance.

EXTERNAL SUPPORT

Children who have little or no external support from home or school are likely to need more direct SALT sessions to make the same amount of progress.

NUMBER OF PRACTICE ITEMS

If the child practises their target stimulus many times during each session, they are likely to need fewer therapy sessions overall. The absolute minimum number of repetitions is 50 per session, but 100+ repetitions are generally recommended.

OPPORTUNITIES FOR PRACTICE

If a child has lots of opportunities for practice and generalisation work, both within the therapy sessions and outside them, progress is likely to be faster and fewer sessions will be needed overall.

CHOSEN THERAPY APPROACH

Different therapy approaches recommend different dosages and it is important to follow the advice given for each approach to maximise the effectiveness.

WHAT IF WE CAN'T OFFER THE RECOMMENDED DOSAGE?

This is a common question that SALTs ask, especially on SSD courses they attend where the dosage recommended is higher than most therapists can provide. Services are beginning to recognise the need for change, especially for children with moderate and severe SSDs; but the reality is that practice often lags behind the evidence, and change is difficult to effect in busy and often already overloaded clinical services. The reasons for being unable to provide frequent sessions usually include a lack of resources in an organisation or, in the case of independent therapists, parents having limited funds for the frequency of therapy recommended. Other reasons include a family's difficulties with attending frequently, for which there may be many valid explanations.

The evidence shows that overall, a higher intensity of sessions is beneficial for most subgroups of children, and that the more severe the child's SSD, the higher the dosage needs to be. However, by reconfiguring the packages of dosage given, it may be possible to deliver differently and improve the speech outcomes for children with SSDs without necessarily having to increase the resources. For example, by increasing the number of repetitions in each session, it may be possible for the child to make the same progress in shorter sessions.

Practical suggestions for reconfiguring sessions include the following:

- Increase the number of repetitions per session by using a chart to ensure 100+ repetitions. Games can be set up for 'little and often' rewards throughout the session for the child (eg, posting a picture for every ten repetitions). Rethink the session structure so that the focus is more on the repetitions, which may mean that playtime/time in between repetitions is reduced. This will facilitate lots of repetitions successively, followed by a quick reinforcer, rather than rewarding each repetition.
- Reorganise sessions so that they are shorter but more frequent (eg, twice a week for 20 minutes rather than once a week for 40 minutes).
- For school-based weekly therapy, see the child for two short sessions on the same day – once in the morning and once in the afternoon.

If therapy cannot be provided at the recommended dosage for the child, this may not be the best time to start therapy for that child. If the prognosis for change with an inadequate level of therapy is no greater than that for no therapy at all, an alternative approach may be considered. Therapists should be aware of the evidence for effective therapy dosage and approach managers and commissioning authorities with the necessary figures. By presenting the evidence in a convincing way, it may be possible to change the funded provision. This particularly applies in the case of children with severe SSDs, such as CAS.

CASE EXAMPLE

Sunil was diagnosed with mild CAS at age five, following several years of relatively unsuccessful intermittent therapy at pre-school age. His areas of need were production of polysyllabic words, as well as some phonological processes (eg, backing). Once he started school, he was able to access therapy from a SALT funded by the school; however, this was only once a week. He needed more frequent sessions, so the timetable was changed so that he could receive shorter but more frequent sessions. The therapist saw him twice each week, on the same day, for 15 minutes; and the teaching assistant also started carrying out daily ten-minute sessions, to carry over the work that the therapist was doing. The teaching assistant was trained to count the number of target words that were elicited so that this was over 100 per session. Sunil progressed much faster than when the sessions were once a week, although the overall direct therapy time remained the same. After two terms of therapy with this revised dosage, his backing had fully resolved and his production of polysyllabic words had reached a level where he only needed occasional reminders in class and at home.

Chapter 37

DISCHARGE: WHEN AND HOW?

REASONS FOR DISCHARGING A CHILD WITH AN SSD

- Speech and language skills are within the normal range for the child's chronological age: This is a common reason for discharge among children with most types of SSDs. However, among the population of children with more complex SSDs – such as CAS, dysarthria, combinations of different types of speech disorders, and additional co-occurring needs – some will never get to the point of having age-appropriate speech. In such cases, children may have residual speech sound distortion or not be fully consistent in their speech. Decisions about discharge can thus be more difficult.
- The parent/child is satisfied with the level of progress: It is always important to consider the feelings of the child and their family when making decisions about discharge. If an older child is happy with their progress and feels positive about themselves and their speech, even if it is not yet age-appropriate, then discharge can be discussed.
- The child is unable to access therapy: This may be due to poor attention, difficulties in engaging with the therapist or one-to-one therapy itself, or another co-occurring factor such as ASD which may affect the child's ability to access therapy that specifically targets CAS. It may be necessary to adjust the focus of the therapy in these cases so that the targets are more communication focused rather than speech focused.

- The child's progress has plateaued: It is important to explore the possible reasons for progress slowing down. Reasons may include reduced motivation in the child or parent or reduced home/school practice in between sessions. It may be that by changing the focus of the therapy, working on new targets, or introducing different motivators, the child's progress may speed up again. It may also be possible that progress has plateaued because the child has genuinely made as much progress as is possible for them at that time. The original speech diagnosis may have been incorrect, and it is worth checking that the type of therapy being given matches the underlying level of impairment if progress has stagnated.
- Non-attendance: This is a controversial reason for discharge and in the UK, there are clearly defined rules for discharge throughout the NHS. Therapists working outside the NHS use their own judgement as to when to discharge for non-attendance; but from a SALT's perspective, it never feels good to discharge a child for this reason, especially when there is a high level of need. It is important that we try to do as much as possible to enable each child to access therapy through whatever means works best for that family. The reasons for non-attendance may relate to difficulties with childcare, transport difficulties, or the family feeling overwhelmed with multiple competing demands. There may also be a language barrier in the case of families who have English as an additional language, and every effort should be made to ensure that these families receive clear, unambiguous appointment letters, phone calls, and emails in their home language, with interpreters used where necessary. Families of all cultures, races, and ethnicities should be given equal access to the SALT service, and this may sometimes require additional time spent explaining how the service operates and how they can access it fully. It may be possible to work through the child's nursery or school to avoid the parents having to take the child to a clinic or the therapist's house if this is particularly difficult for them.

- Limited parental/school involvement to support the therapy programme on a regular basis: Children with SSDs usually make better progress with frequent practice in between sessions, and unfortunately, it may be necessary to pause direct therapy until parental/school support can continue or discharge if this seems unlikely. This decision should always be preceded by efforts to engage with families and/or schools to try to build up support for the child, and discharge should be seen as a last resort.
- Financial limitations: In the independent sector, when parents are funding the therapy themselves, the sad and unfortunate situation may arise in which the family can no longer afford therapy. Some therapists offer a 'pay as you can' service for certain families and this is growing in popularity as the cost-of-living crisis takes its toll. The increasing difficulty in accessing additional support in school for children with severe SSDs means that many children are in a situation where therapy is either unavailable or very limited, so they are turning to the private sector for all their therapy or as a 'top-up'.
- SALT is not the primary area of need: Other areas may need to be addressed before SALT can be continued – for example, where a family needs urgent social care or rehousing, or is going through a breakup or bereavement.
- Maximum potential achieved at the time of the decision: Therapy may not be able to take a child to the level of 100% intelligibility 100% of the time, especially where they have a severe SSD. The child may still struggle with polysyllabic words, new and complex vocabulary, and accurate production in all situations. It may be that one-to-one therapy is no longer moving the child forward with their speech; but some advice to parents and teachers on when and how to correct or prompt in conversation might be the most useful way of continuing to support the child with generalising what they have learned after direct therapy comes to an end.

In some SALT services, older children with SSDs who have already received a period of therapy are discharged if they are unable to produce one or more specific consonants in isolation – particularly if these are later-developing sounds developmentally. The idea behind this decision is that if the child is unable to produce the sound in isolation, there is no point in trying to work on it, especially if they are generally intelligible in conversation. I would suggest, in such cases, that some CV, VC, and CVC work might be valuable, and that it is a shame to 'give up' on certain sounds which the child is very unlikely to develop without SALT support.

Unfortunately, not all therapists are in the position to make their own decisions about when to discharge a child if a discharge policy is in place within that specific SALT service. It is not uncommon for children to be discharged from one SALT service and for parents still to have significant concerns which lead them to refer the child elsewhere to continue the therapy, as discharge criteria vary considerably from one service to another.

In an ideal world, children should have the opportunity to become as proficient at communicating as possible; however, the reality is that resources are limited and tough decisions must be made.

Decisions about discharge should not, however, be the sole responsibility of the SALT but should also involve the opinions of others, so that such decisions are informed by a well-rounded picture of the child from different perspectives. After all, the overall goal of therapy is not for the child to produce perfect speech in front of the therapist in a session, but to communicate successfully with people around them in the real world; to this end, the perspectives of others are important. The psychosocial aspects of a persistent SSD into adulthood should also be considered and addressed; and young adults and their families should be given clear advice about how to access the SALT service at a later stage at the point of discharge.

DISCHARGE OR REVIEW?

In the NHS, it used to be the case that children were put on long-term review – sometimes for years – and the lists of children who had not been seen for a very long time grew to the point where they were unmanageable. More recently, there has been a move towards discharging children if they are not having direct therapy at that time, with the caveat that they may be re-referred later. This has solved the problem of having hundreds of sets of case notes lying dormant without any prospect of the children being followed up. However, it also means that unless parents or schools actively re-refer the child, they may never be seen again and may have a significant SSD which goes untreated. Perhaps we should look towards a compromise: one option to consider is to gradually reduce the session frequency, with increasingly long gaps between each session, as in this way the progress of any residual speech disorder can be tracked more easily. The children who may need direct input at a later stage are thus less likely to be missed.

DISCUSSING DISCHARGE WITH PARENTS/SCHOOLS

Whatever our decisions around discharge or review, parents should be involved at each point of the process. Some may have very strong views about their child remaining on the caseload and this needs careful and sensitive handling, especially if there is a mismatch between the parental expectations from therapy and the reality of the situation.

Schools, too, may need careful and sensitive explanations if they believe that a child whom *they* identify as needing ongoing therapy is felt not to need further input from the therapist.

It may be that the child's needs may be met more effectively by another professional – for example, a dyslexia teacher, clinical psychologist, or special educational needs coordinator (SENCO); however, these decisions require careful explanation and should always be accompanied by a reminder that the child can be referred to SALT later if necessary.

Chapter 38

EFFECTIVE TIME MANAGEMENT

STRESS AND JUGGLING WORKLOADS

Stress at work due to time pressure is a known problem throughout the health and education sectors in particular. We frequently hear about health professionals retiring early or taking time off work with stress-related illness and this seems to be a growing problem. Although the reason that most of us went into SALT initially was to make a significant difference to the lives of people with communication impairments, it is safe to say that the reality of day-to-day life can be far from ideal, in terms of high stress levels and feeling that we're not having a significant impact or can't deliver what we know is needed.

PRACTICAL WAYS TO MANAGE TIME MORE EFFECTIVELY

Rather than trying to fit more activities into less time, it is more helpful to re-evaluate our week and ensure that we examine each aspect of our work so that there is a balance between therapy, admin time, study and learning, support from colleagues, and time for self-care.

Here are some ways to manage time better:

- Schedule in time slots for reading/answering emails – aim for once or twice a day, not all the time.
- Ensure that work which relates to a particular school/clinic is done only on the allocated days, not on other days.
- Complete note-writing on the day of the session; never let it run into the next day.

DOI: 10.4324/9781003480778-43

- Don't feel under pressure to answer messages straightaway.
- Use an organised filing system so that notes are quickly and easily found – for example, different-coloured folders for different schools.
- Never allow sessions to overrun – always stick to the allotted time, even if a family arrives late.
- Don't overpromise and risk underdelivering – for example, only tell a parent that you can print out a lengthy resource for them if you have the time to do this.
- Use e-resources when you can.
- Have a set of portable games on hand for those tricky sessions when you need a quick activity at short notice.
- Always allow turnaround time between sessions to prepare the activities for the next child. Never let other professionals rush you before you're ready.
- Don't be tempted to squeeze in extra sessions or meetings when your diary looks too full.
- Schedule in breaks for drinks, lunch, and planning time.
- Understand that you are working within an imperfect system and be realistic about what is possible.
- Try to finish work on time and don't take it home.
- Know what can be left and what is a priority.
- Build in treats for you and your team, such as lunch out, and social time. This can improve productivity and increase motivation.

There are plenty of excellent courses for SALTs on managing workload and self-care. Supervision is essential for all SALTs and while this is built into NHS roles, independent therapists need to make a conscious decision to source their own supervision. This is an integral part of our work and a professional requirement. Independent therapists can find supervisors who are either SALTs themselves or from another profession. Regular supervision sessions should not just be about clinical work, but our whole working life, including how we are managing stress, work/life balance, and self-care.

Time management is not only about fitting more into a given timeframe, but also about knowing what *not* to do, and how to work more efficiently and productively by having balance in our lives.

Chapter 39

CASELOAD PRIORITISATION

WHERE TO BEGIN?

Large, overwhelming caseloads are commonplace in both the NHS and independent practice. The number of children referred and needing therapy seems to be growing year on year and prioritising children can seem an impossible task. In the NHS, there may be existing prioritisation criteria in operation which may vary according to the specific NHS trust concerned, in which case SALTs may not have the opportunity to make their own decisions about prioritisation. It is helpful to have some broad criteria for prioritisation, provided that there is some wiggle room for flexibility when an individual child has a high level of need for a different reason not specified.

CONSIDER THE FOLLOWING FACTORS ...

- The severity of the SSD and the child's overall intelligibility. Can they communicate their needs? If not, they are at risk of further problems with social interaction and behavioural difficulties.
- Age, attention level, and maturity: Can the child access therapy effectively?
- Hearing status: Can the child hear adequately right now, so that they can access therapy focusing on sounds?
- Is the child frustrated or anxious due to their SSD, or is it affecting their self-esteem?
- Is the child interacting socially with others and can they participate in activities at school that require communication (eg, assemblies, plays, reading aloud, and participating in small group work)?
- Is the child/family motivated to engage fully with therapy?

USE THE ABOVE FACTORS TO DEVISE A POINTS SYSTEM FOR PRIORITISATION

One example of how to consider the above factors is to assign points on a rating scale for each factor, so that the total number of eligibility points can dictate the prioritisation of each child.

For example:

- Intelligibility:
  - Speech is fully intelligible in all contexts – score = 0.
  - Speech is intelligible when context is known – score = 1.
  - Speech is intelligible only to close family – score = 2.
  - Speech is totally unintelligible to other adults and children – score = 3.
- Impact on social interaction:
  - Social interaction with peers appears to be unaffected – score = 0.
  - Social interaction with peers appears to be reduced – score = 1.
  - Social interaction with peers appears to be severely affected by the child's SSD – score = 2.
  - No observable social interaction with others – score = 3.

PROBLEMS WITH USING SET PRIORITISATION CRITERIA

A system which is based on specific criteria must make allowances for children who may score as low priority overall but have a specific need for SALT due to another factor. For example, an older child may be fully intelligible but have a specific articulation disorder which affects them negatively. SALT should never be available only to children who are perceived by others as having a high level of need. Unfortunately, the current system often allows for only the more 'severe' children to receive therapy, leaving those with a 'milder' speech difficulty to access therapy elsewhere or not at all. Many of these children subsequently pop up at a later stage with articulation disorders which may by then be harder to work on, as years of habit have set in.

Therapists are encouraged to make prioritisation decisions in accordance with ethical principles, and especially by looking at the impact on activity and participation.

Chapter 40

GROUP THERAPY

DIFFERENT TYPES

Group therapy may take place at different stages in the therapy process and may include the following:

- Early language/listening and attention groups – these may be for pre-school children who are not yet able to engage with more structured therapy for speech and may be a precursor to further one-to-one therapy later.
- Group work in school for children with SSDs, with a focus on listening and attention skills.
- Group work in schools, run by a teaching assistant or SENCO, for a mixed group of children, all of whom have different types of speech and/or language difficulties.
- Group work in school, run by a teaching assistant, SENCO, or SALT, for children with similar types of speech or language difficulties –for example, children with phonological delay (with either a mixture of delayed processes or just one).

THE ADVANTAGES OF GROUP THERAPY

- More children can be seen at once.
- Therapy sessions can be more frequent – for example, intensive summer holiday groups with daily therapy.
- A greater variety of more interactive and fun activities can be carried out in a group, and groups can be more motivating.
- Children can practise their newly acquired speech skills in the relatively safe environment of a small group of peers.

DOI: 10.4324/9781003480778-45

- Children may feel more comfortable with others who have a similar speech disorder.
- They may benefit from others in the group modelling correct sounds and words.

AND THE DISADVANTAGES ...

- Children may not have the opportunity to practise enough repetitions of the target sounds/words in a group situation.
- Not all SSDs can be treated in a group – for example, CAS has no evidence base to support group therapy.
- Unless a group is homogenous (ie, each child has the same type of speech disorder), it is difficult to target the needs of each child effectively.
- It can be difficult to monitor the progress of each child's speech sounds in a group.

Group therapy is a very useful tool for therapy with SSDs; however, it can rarely replace one-to-one intervention and should usually be used to supplement individual sessions. When groups are run by teaching assistants, these should always be closely monitored by the SALT in terms of the suitability of each child for the group and the targets and activities used in the group. It is never advisable for schools to work on speech with groups of children without the involvement of a SALT.

Chapter 41

BLOCKS AND BREAKS APPROACH

WHAT IS THIS?

The blocks and breaks approach is a very common model for therapeutic intervention – usually not because the evidence says that it is effective, but because it is a convenient way of organising therapy for a large caseload so that lots of children have an opportunity for therapy. The most common model is for a child to have a block of, for example, six sessions, followed by a break of several weeks or months, and then another block of weekly sessions, often with a different set of targets. While that child is having a break, there is thus the opportunity for another child to have therapy during that time. This system is very much based on a model of trying to fit in more children for therapy when time and resources are limited.

Where a blocks and breaks approach is used as the default in an organisation, this means that the individual therapist has limited choices in terms of how to organise their treatment schedule. The RCSLT's 2024 position paper on SSDs recommends that services *not* set a prescribed number of sessions per child, but maintain flexibility in meeting their needs, thus providing a more effective and efficient service. It also specifically states that a six-week therapy block is insufficient to meet the needs of children with SSDs, so we should challenge any attempts to enforce this regime in our organisations.

WHICH GROUPS OF CHILDREN *CAN* BENEFIT FROM THIS APPROACH?

- Children who are working on early listening and attention skills or sound awareness development prior to beginning

more direct speech work may benefit from blocks of group work with breaks in between. Children who are working systematically on a series of different phonological contrasts may have a break after working on and establishing one contrast before moving on the next one. However, it is important that the number of sessions in each block is not rigidly fixed from the outset so that flexibility is maintained.
- Children with phonological delay who are making consistent progress may continue to make progress during a break if natural maturation is also in evidence.
- Children who are participating in a school-based intervention programme will automatically have breaks for school holidays, so there are enforced breaks. This imposed blocks and breaks regime can work well if the therapy is well supported by members of support staff at school during term time. It may be possible to send home activities for parents to practise during the holidays, especially during the long summer break. These should be carefully explained and modelled to the parents, if possible.

WHICH CHILDREN DO *NOT* BENEFIT FROM THIS APPROACH?

- Children with CAS do not benefit from the blocks and breaks approach and therapy can be ineffective if they are given this model of care. All the published programmes for CAS, such as DTTC and the NDP3, recommend ongoing treatment without breaks. One exception is when a child has had a very intensive block of therapy four times a week, in which case a short break of several weeks is recommended.
- Children who are currently working through a series of steps in their therapy programme do not benefit from breaks. Breaks are likely to prolong the whole therapy process and possibly even cause them to regress and forget what they have learned.

AN ALTERNATIVE THERAPY STRUCTURE

If the number of sessions is limited due to organisational constraints, the therapy may be more effective if the sessions offered to the child are shorter but more frequent. Much of the research shows that it is the frequency of sessions, and particularly the number of repetitions of the target word/phrase within each session and overall, which are the most important factors affecting the effectiveness of therapy. It may thus be possible to have the same total amount of therapy time but organise it differently and more effectively so that the child does not have long breaks between treatments.

REFERENCES

RCSLT (2024). New speech sound disorders guidance published. https://www.rcslt.org/news/new-speech-sound-disorders-guidance-published/.

Chapter 42

TELEHEALTH

WHAT IS IT?

Telehealth is the delivery of healthcare where patients and providers are separated by distance. Other terms are sometimes used, such as 'teletherapy', but the RCSLT uses the term 'telehealth' in its 2022 guidance.

Telehealth has been around for several years, particularly in countries where travelling is difficult because of the distances involved, but it wasn't until the Covid-19 pandemic hit in 2020 that this way of working became popular with SALTs in the UK. We were plunged into a situation where we could no longer see children face to face, except in exceptional circumstances, and as a profession we had to be resourceful and find alternative ways of working. SALTs proved themselves to be up to the challenge in these difficult times and developed new ways of working which have changed working practices far beyond the end of the pandemic.

Direct SALT sessions delivered via telehealth have been the subject of many research studies in recent years and the findings are very positive overall for several types of SSDs, especially CAS and articulation disorder.

HOW CAN WE USE IT FOR SSDS?

Telehealth can be used in different ways, including the following:

- Taking case histories at a distance.
- Liaising with parents and/or other professionals through online meetings or sending instructional or information

videos or training materials (known as 'asynchronous telehealth').
- Providing training to parents and others.
- Providing direct therapy to children, either on a one-to-one basis or in groups.

THE ADVANTAGES OF TELEHEALTH

- Therapy can happen over a distance, so we can see children potentially anywhere in the world.
- Parents and children can attend sessions more easily if they have younger siblings to care for or in case of mild illness/inability to drive or travel.
- Some children focus better with screen-based therapy than face to face.
- Sessions can be recorded easily for therapists to watch again at a later stage or for parents to watch to remind them of the strategies they should be using.
- Therapy sessions can take place in different locations – for example, in schools, with teachers and/or teaching assistants present who might be unable to attend a session in person if they had to travel to a clinic or elsewhere.
- The cost of travel (for both therapists and families) is eliminated.
- Increasingly sophisticated features are being developed, so there is a wealth of games and exciting interactive activities which can be used in sessions.
- Telehealth can be used easily for other aspects of the therapeutic process, such as liaison meetings with parents/others, and is especially useful for gathering a group of people together remotely for case discussions.

AND THE DISADVANTAGES ...

- Telehealth relies on a good Wi-Fi signal at both ends if the therapist wishes to carry out a live session with a child. If the signal is poor, it can be very frustrating to have a session cut short or to have poor sound or picture quality.

- The lighting at both ends must be good so that the therapist and child can see each other's faces clearly. It can be difficult to ensure optimal lighting at the child's end in particular, and it can be hard to see the child's articulations clearly.
- The sound quality must be exceptionally good for SSD work, as the perception of sounds by both therapist and child is paramount. This can be difficult to achieve consistently.
- Assessments can be tricky to carry out and most are not standardised for use via telehealth. However, there are some which can be carried out using two devices (either in the same room or remotely), such as the CELF5.
- It can sometimes feel as if there is a lack of connection between therapist and child and between therapist and parent without the face-to-face setting.
- Children with poor listening and attention skills can sometimes find it hard to keep engaged with a telehealth session, especially if they are young.
- There may be issues around social disadvantage where technology is concerned. Telehealth requires the family to have access to suitable technology, which may not be the case for all families. Some sections of the population are more at risk of digital exclusion than others and a particular family's access to technology should be considered before assuming that this is a viable approach.

PREREQUISITES FOR ONLINE THERAPY SESSIONS FOR CHILDREN WITH SSDS

- The child should be able to engage with a screen-based activity for a specific length of time (20-30 minutes) and have sufficient listening and attention skills to sit facing the screen. It may be possible to work remotely with a child who is not yet able to sit on a chair for this length of time by carrying out the session jointly with the parent/teacher. Examples of activities are given in Section 43.

- The parents/school must have an adequate Wi-Fi signal with good sound and picture quality.
- There must always be an adult with the child, preferably visible to the therapist, for safeguarding and safety reasons.

QUICK IDEAS FOR ONLINE THERAPY ACTIVITIES FOR SSDS

- Ask the child to find things in their room beginning with a particular sound.
- Clap out and count syllables using objects in the room or hold up or screenshare pictures.
- Hold up different objects for the child to categorise according to their initial sound. The objects can then be 'eaten' by puppets representing the specific sounds targeted or posted in different boxes.
- Use apps or screenshare games for rhyming and syllable perception.
- Hold up lotto boards with sticky dots (showing pictures beginning with the target sound) and ask the child to name matching pictures which are then stuck onto the board. Magnetic boards can be used in the same way.
- Screenshare pictures for the child to name.
- Use whiteboards and pens as a way of keeping 'score' – for example, add a tick for 't' or 's' when the child names a picture using the correct sound.
- Use emojis as 'stickers' to reward the child as you go along.
- Hold up puppets with movable tongues/lips to show placement for single sounds.
- Use a bag of sound-specific objects for the child to name. A bag with 'cluster' objects or polysyllabic word objects also works well.
- Online sound-loaded pictures and storybooks can be screenshared.
- The drawing facility on different platforms is useful for minimal pair discrimination and production. The child and therapist can take it in turns to draw a spot on the sound they hear at the beginning of the word.

- Use real objects/toys (eg, a toy snake, a ball, a drum) to represent single sounds, as these are more visually appealing on a screen than single-sound pictures.
- Higher-level intelligibility targets for older children can be addressed online using reading or conversation work. Visual cues can be held up by the therapist to prompt the child for appropriate rate, pitch, volume, or clarity (eg, hold up a car for 'too fast' and a snail for 'too slow').
- Keep bubbles and wind-up toys to hand for quick rewards.

Case example

During the Covid-19 pandemic, James' face-to-face therapy sessions had to stop and he started teletherapy sessions instead. This was a totally new experience for him, but it turned out to be something that continued even once lockdown was over.

James had been seen since he was four years old and had a diagnosis of CAS and oromotor apraxia, although he also had features of CPD. At age four, he was unintelligible and using mainly single words, but with age-appropriate comprehension. Direct therapy sessions focused on production of a range of sounds at CVC level, as well as additional work on some specific consonants and vowels which were hard to produce in any word position, and the NDP3 was primarily used. His rate, stress within words, and intonation also needed work.

At age six, James moved to online working, which suited his parents well, as they had recently moved house and their new home was quite far from the therapist's house. A very low-tech approach to therapy was used, which mainly consisted of holding up pictures, but each activity was interspersed with games and 'sticker' emojis were used throughout the session for motivation. Apps were also used, as well as screensharing minimal pair pictures and picture sequences. James continued working through the NDP3 sheets and progressed well through the stages. The work on syllable stress and rate worked well online and as James got older, reading aloud was introduced into the sessions as a way to develop awareness of slowed rate, the importance of pausing at punctuation points, and how to deal with polysyllabic words.

Now age ten, James is fully intelligible, although he still has some inconsistent production of certain sounds and difficulties with polysyllabic words and struggles to control his rate. He continues to have ongoing monthly online sessions to remind him of his strategies and help to support his mum. The online sessions mean that he need not miss school to travel and if any of his siblings is ill, his session is not affected.

While James has not seen a SALT in person for four years, his therapy has continued successfully via telehealth. His family have also received support through the EHCP process and liaison with other SALTs, and school has been facilitated through the use of an online platform.

USEFUL RESOURCES

RCSLT (2022) Telehealth guidance. https://www.rcslt.org/members/delivering-quality-services/telehealth-guidance/

Chapter 43

CONSULTATIVE APPROACH

WHAT IS THIS APPROACH?

The consultative approach includes any kind of intervention which is carried out primarily by parents/carers, teachers, teaching assistants, or other professionals under the guidance of a SALT or SALT assistant. It is specific to one child, where a structured programme is being carried out. The therapist may meet with the adult and/or the child periodically to review progress and reset goals.

In certain parts of the SALT service, the consultative approach has become the most common way of delivering a service to children with SSDs. In some cases, this has been driven by the need to provide a cheap, quick, and easy approach to dealing with an ever-increasing caseload. The reality of the current – and probably ongoing – situation, with too many children referred and not enough therapists or funding available to see them all, means that difficult decisions must be made about the kind of service delivery to use. Unfortunately, there is no evidence to support the use of the 'one size fits all' approach, which in many cases can result in poor progress, demoralised therapists and parents, and ongoing speech difficulties in children for whom a more direct approach would be highly effective.

However, there is real value in the consultative approach for certain groups of children and when it's done well, this method is highly effective. The key, however, lies in the selection of those children who will benefit from this approach and clear knowledge of those who need direct SALT. There has been some valuable research into the progress of children with SSDs using different service delivery models, including working through parents/carers, teachers, teaching assistants, and other professionals.

THE CONCEPT OF A TIERED APPROACH

This model, commonly used in education services, has been used in the speech and language therapy field for several years. Three tiers have been identified, corresponding to the level of need of the child and the type of difficulty present.. SALTs have an important role to play in each tier. The model is based on the principle that the greater the need of the child, the more they will require an increasingly specialised and individualised service:

- Tier 1 – universal: This is a way of providing interventions to *all* children and the role of the SALT is primarily one of training. It may take the form of providing training in schools or nurseries to teaching staff so that they are aware of typical speech development and how they can facilitate the speech development of *all* children in their care, whether those children have an identified SSD or not.
- Tier 2 – targeted: Children with an identified SSD can be targeted by well-supported and highly trained staff, such as teachers and teaching assistants, through groups focused on aspects of communication (eg, listening skills, phonological awareness). These may not necessarily be children who are being seen individually by a SALT but may have been identified by the school as having a level of need.
- Tier 3 – individualised intervention:
  - 3A: This level of intervention is for children with more straightforward, mild difficulties. The intervention can be delivered by others, but managed by a SALT who trains, supports, and monitors those who are carrying out the sessions.
  - 3B: Children with complex or pervasive SSDs (eg, CAS) need individualised intervention from a SALT. They may also be receiving intervention in the other tiers; however, this Tier 3B intervention is essential for their progress.

The 'consultative model' of SALT delivery correlates to Tier 3A in the above list, as this is the tier in which the child has an individualised programme which is delivered by another under the careful supervision of a SALT, who carries out the assessments, sets targets, suggests activities to use, and reviews progress.

This model is very useful for specific groups of children, particularly those with phonological delay or possibly some with CPD. However, there is no evidence that this model is effective with children who have more complex disorders, such as CAS. It may be, however, that other aspects of a child's communication could be addressed using the consultative model (eg, social communication or expressive language development); and it can work well for the SALT to focus on the speech sound aspects while another adult works on other areas of need.

For pre-school children with SSDs who have very little verbal output, the consultative model can work well when used with parents as the main people carrying out the intervention at home, under the guidance of a SALT.

Case example

Jasmine was diagnosed by her school with a phonological delay at age four years, six months. She had several phonological processes, including stopping of fricatives, fronting, and cluster reduction. The SALT visited the school weekly, although the caseload was large and it was not possible to see each child individually. The SALT set targets and gave suggested activities for the teaching assistant to work on with Jasmine, and was available every few weeks for a brief discussion about how the therapy sessions were going. Links to relevant activities were sent to the teaching assistant, as well as recommended apps, which the school purchased. Jasmine made progress over a period of six months and was discharged as her speech was assessed as being age-appropriate.

USEFUL RESOURCES

Ebbels, S, McCartney E, Slonims V, Dockrell J and Norbury C (2019). Evidence-based pathways to intervention for children with language disorders. *International Journal of Language and Communication Disorders,* 54(1), 3-19. This paper explains the tiered model of speech and language therapy intervention.

PART V

THE LINK WITH EDUCATION

Chapter 44

WORKING IN THE SCHOOL SETTING

School-based therapy may take many forms. It may be that a therapist is providing very direct therapy to specific children with SSDs, who may or may not have an EHCP; or they may be responsible for providing a whole-school speech and language therapy service, which requires a greater level of prioritisation and staff training, probably incorporating the tiered approach, as described in section 43.

THE ADVANTAGES OF SCHOOL-BASED THERAPY

- Therapists can observe the child interacting with their peers and teaching staff. This provides valuable information about their communicative confidence in the school setting, attention and concentration skills, and intelligibility. Clinic-based therapy gives only a limited view of how the child interacts, and they may be more confident among their friends or more withdrawn in a whole-class setting. The child can be observed in different settings, such as in the playground, at lunch, at assembly, during PE class, or in free play with peers.
- Development of the child across other areas can be more easily observed in school. Their schoolbooks are accessible and classroom observations can be carried out in, for example, maths or literacy to see how they are progressing in these areas.
- Working in a nursery or other pre-school setting is a particularly effective way to observe a child's global development.

DOI: 10.4324/9781003480778-50

- Access to teachers, teaching assistants, and SENCOs means that liaison is often easier. Therapists can suggest classroom strategies more easily, as they can respond immediately to things that they observe in the classroom, as well as having direct contact with staff members who might be able to carry out work with the child. The tiered approach to therapy delivery is particularly successful when the therapist is based in school.
- Staff members may be able to sit in on therapy sessions and may thus be in a better position to follow up with similar activities, having observed them first hand. Therapists may be able to observe teaching assistants trying out speech activities with a child and can then give relevant feedback and some demonstration/training. This first-hand demonstration is usually far more effective than written advice.
- A greater variety of outcome measures can be used in a school setting – for example, rating the child's intelligibility when talking to peers, their communicative confidence in class, and their anxiety levels when speaking in small groups or to the whole class or school in assemblies or school performances.
- As children with SSDs often have wider difficulties with literacy, memory, social communication, and behavioural dysregulation, these areas can be more easily addressed in the school setting and joint working is easier.
- Children may be happier to engage with therapy sessions in the school setting, as other children will be moving in and out of the classroom to take part in small group or one-to-one interventions of different kinds. They may also focus better at school, as they may see therapy sessions as just another part of their school day when they are required to listen and concentrate.
- From a practical perspective, school-based intervention may work better for parents if they work full time or find it difficult to attend a clinic for any other reason.
- Whole-school training sessions may be arranged so that teachers and support staff can learn strategies to support

all children with SSDs in the classroom setting – for example, by using phonological awareness strategies daily with the whole class and giving appropriate verbal cues to children who are making speech sound errors.

AND THE DISADVANTAGES ...

- Parents are not usually directly involved in the therapy sessions, although in some cases they may be able to come into school to participate in a session. It is thus important to ensure that a system is in place for communicating with parents, whether that is through regular email updates or face-to-face meetings in school.
- Practical arrangements may be tricky – for example, finding a suitable room in which to work, mutually convenient days and times for the therapist to be in school, availability of teaching and support staff to be present in sessions, and adequate time available for staff to liaise and carry out follow-up work.
- There is often a slightly different emphasis between SALTs and teachers – SALTs usually focus primarily on receptive and expressive language, speech, and social interaction, whereas the primary focus of teaching staff is on literacy and academic progress. Although these areas are often interlinked, SALTs and teachers may have different priorities as to which children should be seen for therapy. This may require gentle explanation and training so that each profession develops a fuller understanding of the other.

HOW TO WORK WITH A SCHOOL: TOP TIPS FOR A SUCCESSFUL RELATIONSHIP

- Take every opportunity to speak to staff: Working successfully in school is totally dependent on the level of communication with teachers, teaching assistants, and SENCOs. Otherwise, the school just becomes another clinic space and the rich advantages of working in the school setting are lost. Talk to staff in the corridors, the staff room, over lunch, in the classroom etc, and ensure that they know when you are available for liaison. Ask teachers whether they have noticed any changes in a child's speech sounds, intelligibility, or confidence. Teachers are a valuable source of information about how a child is functioning and interacting in the classroom; together with the therapist's specialist skills, this makes for a team which works well for the good of the child.

- Ensure that you keep up to date with all reports from other professionals, recent assessments, EHCP applications and changes to EHCP arrangements for each child, new diagnoses, new concerns of teachers etc. Schools are such busy places and SALTs may have to chase up these things; otherwise, important changes may occur without the therapist's knowledge.
- Be very organised with arranging room bookings, checking on dates when children may not be in school or may have unavoidable things happening in school such as sports day, performances, or test week. Ensure that there is a named person at school who is responsible for informing the SALT if a child is absent on the day of their session.
- Provide specific links to therapy resources or lend games and activities to be carried out at school. Teaching and support staff rely on and are highly appreciative of our suggestions and activities, and rarely have the time to create their own activities on top of their other demands.

WORKING WITH TEACHING ASSISTANTS

Working with teaching assistants can be an excellent way of helping children to progress faster with their speech. Teaching assistants can be trained to carry out effective work with children, provided that they have observed the therapist first and have clear instructions as to how to carry out the activities. Depending on the needs of the specific child, a teaching assistant may be able to carry out speech activities effectively, as well as monitoring the child's progress. The more severe or complex the child's speech, the more frequent the contact with the SALT will need to be.

Here are some examples of different models of SALT/teaching assistant therapy:

- Phonological delay: If a child has a common phonological process (eg, fronting or stopping), the teaching assistant may be able to carry out some targeted phonological work following the SALT's programme for the child. It is important for the teaching assistant to know the level at which to begin the work (eg, the discrimination stage or the single-word production stage), and to be aware of whether there are any difficulties with the child articulating the sound in isolation. If the child is unable to produce a particular sound in isolation (eg, /k/), it is often helpful for the SALT to work on production of this until the child can use it in CVs and VCs, and then to pass on the child to the teaching assistant to continue from this point.

  If the child has just one delayed phonological process, an experienced teaching assistant may be able to work on this for several weeks or a term without the SALT being involved, unless there are any specific difficulties.

  Group work or paired work is also very useful for teaching assistants to do with children who have similar types of phonological delay, and this can be highly effective. Larger primary schools are likely to have several children who have similar types of phonological delay who may be able to work well in a group, using similar activities.
- Articulation disorder: A child with a difficulty in producing a specific speech sound(s) accurately (where that sound would normally have been present at the relevant age) may need some direct articulation work with the SALT; but once they have begun to produce the sound in isolation and in syllables, the teaching assistant may be able to continue generalisation work so that the child can begin using the new sound in different syllable positions, in longer words, and then in phrases and sentences. Again, many teaching

assistants have the skills to carry out this type of work with minimal support from the SALT.

- CPD: As with children who have phonological delay, teaching assistants may be able to carry out direct sessions with these children, probably on a one-to-one basis rather than in groups, as their speech patterns are likely to be very different. The SALT will need to identify the exact speech patterns and then give the teaching assistant specific targets and suggested activities to work on.
- IPD: As these children need a different type of therapy, teaching assistants will need to observe the SALT's sessions and work much more closely with them if CVI is being used. Again, one-to-one sessions rather than group sessions will be necessary, alongside the parents carrying over the speech work at home daily. More frequent liaison between the teaching assistant and the SALT will be needed for children with these inconsistent disordered patterns.
- CAS: It is not advised for teaching assistants to work independently with children with CAS; however, if specific areas need additional practice – for example, production of polysyllabic words, other aspects of the child's speech (eg, additional phonological areas), or generalisation work – this may work well.

As with most children with SSDs, their difficulties are unlikely to fall neatly into one single category and teaching assistants may be able to work on the less complex aspects with less supervision needed.

Also, as many children with SSDs have other areas of communication which require intervention (eg, language, phonological awareness, or social communication), these are areas on which the teaching assistant may be able to work, while the SALT focuses on the more complex aspects of the SSD.

Teaching assistants are an extremely valuable resource in schools and have a key role to play in enabling SALTs to carry out therapy programmes with many children on their caseload.

Case example

Jenn is a teaching assistant in a mainstream primary school who has a child of her own with an SSD. This has given her additional insight into the different ways of working with children with SSDs, having been through the speech and language therapy process herself. Jenn was asked to become the specialist teaching assistant for speech and language in the school and the SALT was asked to train her up. This required lots of time to teach her the basics of how SALTs assess and treat different types of communication difficulties, as well as to attend some online courses designed for teaching assistants. Jenn started by observing lots of therapy sessions; after a term, she was able to take on a caseload of children herself – mainly those with language delay and delayed phonology. She built up a resource kit with games and activities for different speech sound substitutions, especially the more common ones, and was then able to use these for group and paired work. This meant that the SALT saw only those children with more complex disorders, while Jenn saw those with a 'delay', alongside termly liaison with the SALT to discuss their progress.

Chapter 45

EHCPS AND REPORT-WRITING

WHERE ARE WE AT WITH SEND SUPPORT FOR CHILDREN WITH SSDS?

In 2022, the Department of Health recognised that change is needed in the system, as the necessary outcomes were not being met. The RCSLT and the Association of Speech and Language Therapists in Independent Practice (ASLTIP) responded and commented that we need:

- More jointly funded commissioning between health and education.
- *Early* intervention for children to reduce the impact of communication needs when children are older.
- Adequate and timely support to children without necessarily needing an EHCP.
- A consistent joined-up approach so that SALT support is easily accessible.

However, change is slow and there may be situations in which the imperfect system limits our ability to provide what is needed to children with SSDs.

THE PURPOSE OF A SALT REPORT

Where a child has a severe SSD, either in isolation or co-existing with other difficulties, and a school, nursery, or parent is applying for additional funding through an EHCP, SALTs are usually asked to provide a report as part of the statutory assessment. The aim of the report is to describe the child's needs and how their communication and education are impacted by the SSD, and to provide recommendations about what SALT input

DOI: 10.4324/9781003480778-51

and support in the classroom are necessary. If the parents and/or school feel that the child is unable to access education in a mainstream class, the EHCP will need to justify why this is the case and recommend the type of placement which is required (eg, a specialist language unit). There is a move to reduce the number of EHCPs for children and try to find other ways of providing the necessary support for them; however, there is significant variation throughout the country and each local education authority (LEA) has a slightly different way of approaching this.

The current situation can be challenging for parents, schools, and other professionals, and there are often delays and differences of opinion between LEAs and those who know the child which can result in incorrect placement and/or insufficient support being given to the child initially.

The LEA may turn down an application for a statutory assessment at the initial application stage, for a variety of reasons – often because insufficient evidence or information has been submitted. At this early stage, it is important for parents and professionals to build a strong case with detailed evidence of what measures have been put in place and how the child has responded to these. If the LEA believes that the child is making sufficient progress with the current level of support, there is not a strong case for an EHCP.

WHAT TO INCLUDE IN AN EHCP REPORT

If asked to provide a report as part of the statutory assessment process, there are different formats and guidelines which SALTs can use, and different NHS trusts and organisations may have their own specific format. However, the following sections are often included:

- A summary of the child's speech, language, and communication needs.
- Background information:
  - Date of referral.
  - Reason for referral.

- Provision received to date.
- Summary of needs.
- Description of the child's current speech, language, and communication skills:
  - Attention and listening skills.
  - Receptive language.
  - Expressive language.
  - Speech sounds.
  - Social interaction skills.
- Summary and recommendations:
  - Therapy goals.
  - Long term.
  - Medium term.
  - Short term.
  - Recommended SALT provision over the next 12 months.
  - Recommended educational support.
  - Specific setting recommendations.

It is particularly important to be specific about the child's speech and language needs and how they impact on functioning in areas such as literacy, phonological awareness, ability to access whole class learning, intelligibility, social interactions, self-esteem, and social participation. If the child requires AAC, this should be explained in detail, with what is needed and the costings specified. SALT provision should include details such as the following:

- Who should carry out the input (eg, SALT/teaching assistant/combination)?
- How frequent should the sessions be?
- How many sessions should there be throughout the year?
- How much staff liaison/training by the SALT is needed?
- How much time is needed for assessments, writing up notes, planning, attending annual review meetings, writing reports, liaising with others etc?

It is important to focus on the child's level of *need* rather than allowing our recommendations to be driven or limited by the *available resources.* This has been an ongoing difficulty for many years in the system, although the RCSLT is clear about the centrality of a child's *needs* when recommending and implementing speech and language therapy for children with SSDs.

WHEN MORE THAN ONE SALT IS CONTRIBUTING TO AN EHCP

When more than one SALT is involved with a child, especially if an EHCP application is being made, frequent and effective communication between the therapists is particularly important. This should reduce the risk of the SALTs producing reports which recommend totally different levels of input for the child. Even if there is good communication, however, therapists may still have a difference of opinion, which can cause difficulties and confusion for parents and LEAs.

One difficulty is where NHS trusts are allowed only to recommend one of a specific number of 'packages of care' in an EHCP report, which often refers to a fixed number of sessions per year, without allowing for an individual therapist to tailor the therapy package to the individual child. For example, some NHS trusts will only recommend six, 12, or 18 sessions per year for a child in a mainstream class. This equates to a maximum of one session every two weeks, which is seriously inadequate for a child with a severe SSD. Careful, tactful negotiation between both therapists is the only way forward in these situations. However, the reality is that some children will never have EHCPs with adequately funded SALT provision and parents may be forced to pay for additional therapy, if they can.

There are currently particular difficulties in certain areas of the UK where LEAs may only accept the advice of NHS SALTs, rather than independent SALTs, although this is currently being challenged by the RCSLT and is in a state of flux. In October 2024, ASLTIP released a statement addressing concerns about LEAs refusing to consider reports from independent SALTs as part of the EHCP process. This statement emphasises that all practising SALTs should meet the same professional standards and have a shared commitment to children's needs. It calls for fair treatment and recognition of the work of independent SALTs as part of the EHCP process, as mandated by the SEND Code of Practice. It is hoped that this statement may prompt a paradigm shift in how NHS and independent SALTs are viewed by LEAs: they can contribute equally to the EHCP process and should have equal recognition.

Chapter 46

SEND TRIBUNALS

WHEN MIGHT A CASE COME BEFORE A TRIBUNAL?

Sometimes a draft EHCP requires amendment if it does not appear to specify the correct level of support needed or if the setting is felt to be incorrect. Parents have the opportunity to appeal any LEA decision and there is a process for doing this. However, sometimes the LEA turns down an appeal and parents may consider taking the case to a tribunal. SEND tribunals are very much a last resort for parents and, from a SALT perspective, may take place for any of the following reasons:

- The LEA has decided not to give the child an EHCP and the amount of funding available in the school does not cover the level of SALT/teaching assistant sessions which the child needs.
- The LEA has awarded an EHCP, but the provision is felt to be inadequate (eg, fortnightly rather than weekly therapy funded).
- The EHCP names an educational setting which is felt to be inappropriate for the child's needs (eg, a mainstream school as opposed to a specialist language unit).
- The EHCP specifies the provision accurately, but it is not being implemented by the school in practice (eg, the EHCP states that daily carryover work by a teaching assistant is needed, but this is not taking place).

The purpose of a SEND tribunal is to overturn the decision of the LEA by demonstrating that the initial decision was incorrect.

WHAT HAPPENS IN A SEND TRIBUNAL?

The 'parties' at the tribunal are the parents and the LEA. The LEA gives evidence as to why it believes its decision is correct, in terms of the decision being in the best interests of the child. The parents and (usually) the school give their evidence as to why they believe the LEA's decision is incorrect and what support they believe the child needs. Usually, the parents and school are of the same view, although this is not always the case; and it may happen that the school agrees with the LEA decision, but the parents disagree. Both sides may avail of expert witnesses, who are answerable to the tribunal and not to the side who has enlisted them.

THE SALT'S ROLE IN TRIBUNALS

A SALT may be asked by the LEA or the parent to assess the child, write a report, and possibly attend the tribunal itself. The SALT is acting as an *expert witness* and is not, strictly speaking, *representing* the parents or the child, but simply using their specialist knowledge and expertise to give evidence which supports their decisions about speech and language therapy needs, recommendations, and provision for the child. The evidence should be totally unbiased and should not be affected by parental pressure or other factors, even if the parents are commissioning the SALT. All aspects of the advice should be justifiable and supported by evidence, quoting specific research where appropriate, as this will strengthen the case for ensuring that a specific dosage, therapy type, and level of expertise (eg, a qualified and specialist SALT in SSDs) are granted. It is thus essential that SALTs who undertake tribunal work always act within the limits of their knowledge, skills, and experience, and do not undertake this role if they are not fully equipped to do so. If two or more SALTs are involved with the child, a lead therapist should be identified who can take responsibility for communicating effectively and liaising with the LEA.

There are some excellent training courses available for SALTs who are interested in developing the necessary skills in medico-legal work, tribunals, and report-writing for expert witnesses.

HOW TRIBUNAL REPORTS DIFFER FROM EHCP REPORTS

Tribunal reports (known as 'expert witness reports') are usually much more detailed than EHCP reports and should be written in a specific format. However, there are some similarities between the two types of reports – for example, the need to recommend speech and language therapy support according to the child's *needs*, rather than the *available resources*. In tribunal reports, it is important that the SALT writing it demonstrates how their specialist knowledge, experience, and expertise qualify them sufficiently to make appropriate recommendations for that child.

SUGGESTED FORMAT FOR TRIBUNAL REPORTS

- Introduction:
  - The purpose of the report.
  - Who commissioned it.
  - The experience and specialist knowledge of the author, particularly with reference to SSDs.
  - The documents seen and when they were written.
- Part 1 – background history:
  - A summary of the case history, including SALT involvement.
- Part 2 – identification and summary of speech and language therapy needs:
  - An evaluation of the child's needs based on a comprehensive, broad-based, up-to-date assessment of all areas of communicative functioning and, where possible, in a range of contexts.
  - Summaries of previous therapy – a description of progress over time and strategies and support provided.
  - A statement of the SALT's involvement with the child, including for how long, and how the child's needs and

progress are being monitored in school. The source of any observations or information given in the report should be clarified – for example, whether the information was gained through first-hand observation by the SALT or reported by others.
- An analysis of the child's speech, language, and communication. Evidence should include clinical observation alongside informal and formal assessments, where possible, to support statements about the child's difficulties and rate of progress. The choice of assessments should be explained and the results evaluated.
- An explanation of the implications of the described difficulties in relation to the child's educational setting – particularly the impact on the child's social participation, learning, and ability to access the curriculum.
- Information on how the child is functioning in their educational placement, including a description of how and where the child works best and a broad description of the speech, language, and communication outcomes being sought for the child.

- Part 3 – provision:
  - Facilities (eg, what type of room is required).
  - Modifications (eg, use of alternative or augmentative communication).
  - Resources (eg, provision of high-tech communication software).
  - Staff knowledge and skills – the level of experience that teaching staff should have.
  - The SALT provision needed to train staff to provide a supportive and inclusive environment.
  - The resources and features needed for the SALT programme to be effective.
  - The model of therapy provision chosen, with a clear rationale for this.
  - The projected outcomes, including reference to research data.
  - Models of intervention (some are described here, but others can be used):

- Supported inclusion of the child – this will usually involve a specified number of SALT hours for joint planning, co-working, and training sessions to enable school staff to make teaching style changes or environmental changes to optimise the inclusion of the child in the classroom.
- Child skill development through inclusive means – the SALT will support the school staff to carry out work with the whole class or in small groups to develop targeted language or communication skills. A specific number of hours will be needed for meeting planning, demonstration, and preparation.
- Child skill development through the integration of individualised targets – the SALT will work with parents and staff members to integrate individualised targets into daily life at school and home.
- Child skill development through individualised programmes of work – the SALT will provide a regular programme of individualised intervention which should be outlined in detail and should relate directly to the child's needs as described in the report. The number of hours per year should be specified. The person or people who will be carrying out the work should be specified (eg, SALT, SALT assistant, teaching assistant). If anyone other than a SALT is carrying out the work, they should have the knowledge, skills, and experience to do so. The number of hours specified should also include time for preparation, demonstration, discussion, observation, monitoring of implementation, progress reviews, and measurement of outcomes.
- Children requiring regular and continuing speech and language therapy – while direct interventions are part of a wider package, these may change over time with evolving levels of need, so flexibility is needed.

- Part 4 – placement:
  - A description and rationale for a type of placement which follows on from the evidence gained from the assessment in Part 2 and the provision outlined in detail in Part 3. A specific school should not be named at this stage; however, a parent or LEA may ask a SALT that they have commissioned to comment on a type of placement in a specific school in terms of suitability and this may be presented orally at a tribunal hearing.

The SALT recommendations throughout should be **specific**, **quantifiable**, and **flexible**.

USEFUL RESOURCES

Expert witness training is available through Bond Solon and is suitable for SALTs who are interested in this area of work. See www.bondsolon.com for details.

Chapter 47

THE LINK WITH LITERACY

The association between CPD and IPD, phonological awareness, and literacy (reading and spelling) is well documented. If we identify phonological awareness deficits, we must address these as well as expressive phonology, so that children with SSDs do not remain at additional risk of literacy difficulties. It has been shown that where a child has an SSD lasting beyond eight years, this has a negative impact on educational attainment in English, maths, and science, which continues into secondary school.

STAGES OF LITERACY DEVELOPMENT

Theories of early reading development identify the following phases:

- Logographic phase: Children can recognise a limited number of words by recognising prominent visual features.
- Alphabetic phase: Children have acquired some letter-sound knowledge and have started using alphabetic information systematically to support reading and spelling attempts. Children cannot move through this phase without the development of phonological awareness, alongside the integration of this and phonics knowledge when they attempt to read and write.
- Orthographic phase: This is the most advanced phase, during which children learn to recognise larger word segments automatically. Grapheme-phoneme conversion for each letter is no longer necessary, although children may have to use this strategy at times for unfamiliar or trickier words.

WHICH CHILDREN WITH SSDS ARE AT RISK OF LITERACY DIFFICULTIES?

Children with a history of SSDs are at greater risk of literacy impairment; however, certain groups of children within the umbrella of SSDs have significantly increased risk. These groups include the following:

- Children who still have signs of an SSD at the start of formal literacy teaching (in the UK, this is around the age of four or five). Those whose SSD has resolved by this time are at minimal risk of literacy difficulties.
- Children with phonological awareness difficulties (with or without an associated SSD).
- Children with combined language and speech difficulties at the age of formal literacy teaching.
- Children with SSDs who have *atypical* speech errors.
- Children who have low non-verbal cognition and/or a family history of dyslexia.

The common factor in these groups which have a higher risk of literacy difficulties appears to *phonological awareness* difficulties, which are more likely if a child has consistent use of typical and atypical phonological patterns. The children who have a lower risk of literacy difficulties are generally those with inconsistent phonological disorder and articulation disorder, provided that they do not also have other risk factors.

LITERACY DEVELOPMENT IN SSDS

Children need access to well-specified phonological representations for both speech accuracy and phonological awareness. These phonological representations store phonological information about words in long-term memory, so any disruption to the accurate formation of the representations, their storage, or their retrieval is likely to result in speech production difficulties and problems with phonological awareness. Children with difficulties in these areas are thus at greater risk of literacy difficulties. SSDs can affect both the rate and the accuracy of literacy acquisition.

This complex relationship between phonological awareness, phonological representations, speech production, and literacy development means that we need to look out for any red flags that might indicate that a child has, or is at significant risk of, literacy difficulties at school.

It is not only at the single-word level that children with SSDs may have difficulties with reading and spelling, but also at higher levels of reading, such as reading text for comprehension tasks or understanding a story or worksheet in class. These areas are often highlighted by teachers when children have progressed further in school, even if the child has mastered the basic stages of learning to read. There is evidence that literacy can be impacted into the teenage years, especially as the demands on literacy are much greater: writing essays, critically evaluating a piece of research, forming an argument, dealing with more complex and technical vocabulary, and structuring written work in different ways, such as presenting posters or using PowerPoint.

THE SALT'S ROLE IN LITERACY DEVELOPMENT

Although many children with SSDs have an increased risk of literacy difficulties, we are not the sole professionals to work in this area. We need to be clear about the boundaries of our role, ensuring that we don't become the professionals to whom schools turn for any child who is struggling to read and spell. This is particularly important if we are asked to work with a child who is slow to learn to read but has no sign of an SSD and whose other communication skills are age appropriate. There may be other reasons for their difficulties with reading and we are not usually the appropriate professionals to work on literacy in such cases. Also, children who have an articulation disorder, age-appropriate phonological awareness skills, but delayed literacy development are also not children for whom literacy should be our focus. It is important that we discuss this with teachers so that they have a clear understanding of the scope of our work and when they should enlist the help of another professional, such as a specialist dyslexia teacher or teaching assistant.

Children whom we identify as having a phonological awareness difficulty as well as an SSD can certainly receive input from us in this area and Section 30 describes some ways in which we can implement phonological awareness intervention, particularly working with schools to support this. Working on phonological awareness is also likely to effect change in speech production and literacy, so this is a key area to target if it has been identified as an area of need.

There are some children whom it is entirely appropriate to work with on literacy skills – particularly those with a language disorder who have difficulties with reading comprehension and/or formulating their written answers in these tasks, and those who find it hard structuring written work for stories, sequencing written instructions, and writing essays. Our work with these children can extend throughout the secondary school years – particularly if they are in specialist language settings, have an EHCP in a mainstream school, or need additional support with university or job applications.

Case example

Matt was seven years old and had never been referred to a SALT. His school was concerned about his spelling of words with 'r', 'w', 'l', and 'y', and he appeared to struggle to know when to use each of these letters in his written work. Assessment showed that he also had some articulation and phonological errors with this group of sounds, as well as considerable difficulties with phonological awareness – particularly in identifying initial and final consonants. He had some one-to-one speech and language therapy to work on his articulation of 'l' and 'r' in words and phrases, as well as some phonological awareness work. He progressed significantly with his production; however, his spelling and phonological awareness remained a concern, and the SALT recommended referral for a diagnostic dyslexia assessment. This resulted in a diagnosis of dyslexia at age eight, and he was discharged from speech and language therapy and began receiving specialist dyslexia teaching in school.

PART VI

CONCLUDING THOUGHTS

Chapter 48

THE CONCEPT OF 'DISORDER'

Our understanding and use of terminology in the field of medicine has changed beyond recognition in the last 100 years. The medical model, developed in the 18th century, focuses heavily on the concept of 'disorder' and 'impairment', with the implication that people who deviate from the 'norm' need to be 'treated' so that they become like everyone else.

THE IMPORTANCE OF TERMINOLOGY

The social model presents a different perspective, highlighting the societal barriers which discriminate against certain groups of people. Taking this one step further, the neurodiversity paradigm, developed in the 1990s, recognises the whole diversity of the mind-body experience. For example, there has been a shift towards respecting differences rather than viewing aspects of behaviour and communication in children with autism as 'disordered'. This shift has resulted in lots of new terminology to describe people who think or interact with the world around them in different ways. People who have ASD, ADHD, dyslexia, or dyspraxia are often referred to as 'neurodivergent'; and terms such as 'impairment', 'defect', 'incompetence', and 'deficiency' are becoming less common in many parts of the world due to their negative and static quality. They are often replaced by more neutral terms, such as 'difference' or 'barrier'. 'Neurodiversity-affirming language' and an approach to therapy which recognises differences in the way that different people use their brains value, respect, and support each person's unique personality, differences, and preferences, rather than viewing the person as needing 'fixing' or as 'impaired'.

DOI: 10.4324/9781003480778-55

The use of different terminology can affect how children view themselves and how professionals view the children with whom they work. The language that we use has the power to hurt or to boost a person; to criticise or empower.

APPLICATION TO SSDS

Although we use the term 'disorder' in the diagnostic label 'speech sound disorder', this is not intended to be negative or judgemental, but simply to reflect the significant impact that this can have on a child and the need for intervention.

However, with SSDs, it is important to distinguish between features in a child's speech which affect intelligibility (and thus the success or otherwise of communication) and those which are more to do with the 'acceptability' of the child's speech sounds. Intelligibility is significantly affected by vowel distortion, inconsistency, and suprasegmental features such as rate and prosody. However, a child who has one or two consistent articulatory substitutions which do not have phonological consequences (eg, a lateral 's' or labiodental 'r'), in the absence of other unusual speech features, is unlikely to have intelligibility issues. We could thus question whether there is justification for working on these areas.

Decisions such as these are affected by how the child feels about their speech, their age, and any emotional impact on them. However, we could argue that the problem is with the way in which society views speech which is in any way different. Unconscious bias is strongly embedded in society and listeners can be swayed by accent, level of fluency, rate or volume of speech, overall clarity, and other speech features which can influence the listener's views about the speaker's intellectual level, social class etc. These preconceptions and biases can have a negative outcome for the speaker.

There has been an increase in public awareness about different types of communication differences – particularly in the field of stammering, where celebrities who stammer have helped to raise the profile and public understanding of dysfluency. CAS has also been discussed openly on social media and some young people have huge followings due to their posts about their experiences of CAS.

Societal views change very slowly, but in time I hope that we will move towards becoming a society that embraces different ways of speaking, while also supporting the valuable interventions which are needed to help so many children become more intelligible and confident communicators in every aspect of their lives.

Chapter 49

WHERE WE ARE HEADING WITH SSDS

NEW TREATMENT APPROACHES

New interventions are continually being trialled and it can be hard to keep abreast of what is coming out of the many studies which are underway. One way is to use Google Scholar to check for new interventions; by doing this frequently, we can keep up with what is happening worldwide in the field of SSDs.

More recent approaches include a renewed interest in motor learning theory and its application to SSDs, particularly CAS; and the DTTC intervention, devised by Professor Edythe Strand in the US, which has gained popularity in the UK. Strand's online training videos and in-person masterclasses have trained a growing number of SALTs to a high level to implement this highly effective treatment with children who have the most severe SSDs.

High-tech therapies are also developing rapidly. The emerging evidence base for biofeedback interventions (mainly single case studies and single case experimental designs) points towards the effectiveness of these methods. Acoustic biofeedback uses either a spectrogram or a linear predictive coding spectrum to distinguish speech sounds.

A variety of apps are also available for use in therapy and new ones are being developed all the time. Two which are particularly popular with SALTs are Articulation Station Hive and Articulation Arcade (available via the App Store), both of which have a large database of pictures beginning with all sounds in each word position, which can also be used for phrase and sentence work, as well as minimal pair activities.

USE OF AI

In recent years, an increasing number of research studies have explored the use of AI in the field of speech and language therapy, including in relation to SSDs. Many have focused specifically on therapy with children who have articulation disorders – particularly on the use of automated AI tools which are capable of ASR and can give children specific feedback based on their production attempts. Studies have not yet compared the outcomes of AI-based automated therapy with those of direct therapy with a SALT; however, many studies have shown significant progress, particularly with articulation disorders and the use of AI to increase the frequency of speech practice in between direct therapy sessions. Its use in geographical areas where therapy provision is limited has also been proposed in many studies.

AI is currently generating considerable interest among SALTs both in clinical practice and in research. Potential uses for therapists include the following:

- To help with day-to-day tasks such as creating therapy resources (eg, ask ChatGPT or another AI chatbot to generate a series of CVC pictures for 'p' words, write a story with lots of 'l' words for a child who loves dinosaurs, or create a matching game with polysyllabic words which are key terms for GCSE chemistry).
- To handle administrative tasks such as generating information packs and handouts, creating resources for training others, finding references, and designing case history forms and policy documents.
- As a high-tech AAC aid for children who require a sophisticated system which can recognise their speech (which may be partially unintelligible to others) and then generate an intelligible version for the listener.
- For AI-based automated therapy – the child is trained to use a mobile or computer-based application which can recognise their speech differences and give feedback (visual, pictorial, auditory, or a combination), so that they can

practise their target sounds or words without the need for a therapist or parent to work with them directly. This can be used to supplement the child's face-to-face therapy, enabling them to have additional practice in the week.

There is also ongoing research into the possibility of using AI for the whole process of assessment, diagnosis, therapy goal-setting, and treatment for children with SSDs. However, it is extremely unlikely that AI will ever be able to replace SALTs, as the skills involved in the therapeutic process – from initial referral to discharge – are more complex, far-reaching and involved than an AI system could possibly deliver. Building therapeutic relationships over time with children, their families, and their schools, and analysing speech in terms of combining auditory skills, observation, and case history information to build a case profile, are skills unique to SALTs. Concerns have also been raised over data confidentiality issues, which will need to be addressed.

However, AI is very much here to stay and advances in the quality of speech recognition mean that in future, this may become a highly effective tool in our toolkit for the assessment and treatment for children with SSDs.

SERVICE DELIVERY ISSUES

The challenges of delivering an effective service to children with limited resources remain ever-present and the situation shows no signs of improving. The solution lies in collecting and providing evidence to commissioners that the speech and language therapy service is effective and efficient. This requires the systematic collection of outcome data and two methods are currently being used to achieve this:

- ROOT: This online tool of the RCSLT supports SALTs with collecting and collating data on therapy outcome measures.
- Maximising the Impact of Speech and Language Therapy for Children with Speech Sound Disorders (known as the MISLToe study): This study aims to:

- Carry out an umbrella review of existing evidence.
- Conduct workshops with SALTs and parents to identify the processes through which children with SSDs are assessed and diagnosed in NHS services (which will lead to an agreed process for SSD diagnosis).
- Present the results of the review, workshops, and surveys for discussion by an expert panel.

A follow-on study will focus on establishing a process for the collection of a large dataset which can be used to answer many questions on SSDs and compare outcomes across different care pathways.

Through these types of data collection and analysis, we hope to be able to demonstrate the types of interventions which work and the subgroups of children who respond to different interventions. This should assist in identifying the areas that need additional resources. Also, if we can demonstrate the effective use of SALT assistants and teaching assistants in SSD interventions, this will show that efficiency measures have been taken.

APPS FOR SPEECH SOUND WORK

- Articulation Arcade: https://www.aptus-slt.com
- Articulation Station Hive: https://apps.apple.com

USEFUL RESOURCES

ChatGPT. https://chatgpt.com
Google Scholar. https://scholar.google.com
RCSLT. Outcome measures. https://www.rcslt-root.org

Chapter 50

MOVING FORWARD WITH CONFIDENCE

PERSONAL GOALS AND SUPERVISION

In supervision sessions, we should be thinking about setting and evaluating personal goals – both those which are directly clinically based and those which relate to our career development. The HCPC is clear that supervision sessions should be led by the supervisee, rather than treating these sessions as a time to discuss cases (clinical case discussion can perhaps take place in another context). However, clinical cases and questions about specific children may well be at the forefront of our minds, and it may be that recurring patterns and themes arise in our clinical life which can be explored in a supervisory conversation.

Questions to ask ourselves include the following:

- What events/conversations have made me stop to think?
- Have I wondered whether there might have been a different way of approaching the situation?
- What events/conversations have caused me to worry afterwards?
- Have I had new ideas and/or thoughts about developing or enhancing my skills? If so, what have I done about them?
- Am I moving forward or staying in the same place in terms of my clinical work and other aspects of my working life?
- What is stopping me from moving forward?

In the field of SSDs, specific questions to ask ourselves on a regular basis include the following:

- How am I assessing, treating, and managing my caseload of children with SSDs?
- Am I clear about differentially diagnosing different subtypes of children with SSDs?
- Am I keeping up to date about new treatment methods which are being developed?
- Am I using the updated clinical guidance and information on SSDs from the RCSLT?
- Which assessment and/or treatment methods do I need to learn more about?
- Am I using a variety of therapy approaches with my caseload of children with SSDs or sticking to those with which I am familiar?
- How am I putting into practice any new approaches that I have learned through courses, workshops, online learning etc?
- How am I explaining my clinical decision-making to parents and others?
- Am I continually re-evaluating my practice?

If we ask ourselves these questions regularly – perhaps every six months – we are unlikely to become stale with our therapy and are more likely to use evidence-based practice and continually hone our clinical decision-making skills.

CHALLENGING BARRIERS TO BEST PRACTICE

The RCSLT encourages us to challenge structures, systems, or therapy delivery models which we believe are barriers to best practice. This may be very difficult to do in the workplace, but we have a personal and professional responsibility to provide the very best standards of care to all the children and families we work with.

SELF-CARE

This is a sometimes-overused term in our society, but it is key if we are to become effective practitioners. It involves ensuring that we have balance in every aspect of our lives and are not slavishly meeting the demands of others around us to the detriment of our own mental, physical, or psychological health. We need to be decisive and intentional in our efforts to spend time wisely, so that we give ourselves due care and attention. If we don't look after ourselves, we are unlikely to be able to give the best possible service to the children and families with whom we work. Too much time is lost through work-related stress and burnout, but there are some strategies that we can put into practice to reduce the risk of this happening. These include:

- Scheduling in specific time for relaxation, exercise, lunch breaks, and social time.
- Ensuring that the professional demands and expectations of us do not exceed our capacity to deal with them.
- Knowing when and how to say 'no'.
- Having good supervision in place.
- Not overpromising when we know that this might increase our stress levels to unacceptable levels.
- Not always aiming for perfection – no one can achieve this.
- Accepting that we can make mistakes and learn from them.
- Asking for help or support as soon as we recognise that we need it.
- Not always replying to emails or messages straightaway but scheduling in set times to read and respond to them.
- If a session does not seem to have gone well, trying to find something positive in it and knowing that every SALT has good and not so good sessions.
- Ensuring that each day has a moment of joy: a coffee shop visit, time with a good book, or meeting a friend.
- Remembering and saying out loud to ourselves, 'I can do this; I've got this' if we feel inadequate.
- Remembering that SALTs are the communication specialists and, particularly with SSDs, no other professionals are equipped to do this job.

STEPPING OUT OF OUR COMFORT ZONE

To be highly motivated, forward-thinking professionals who are actively engaged in lifelong learning and striving for best practice requires us to be brave and to step out of our comfort zone. This may involve taking on a new challenge, such as researching a new therapy approach and sharing it with our team or learning a new therapy technique that we are unfamiliar with; taking a totally new turn in our career path, such as working towards specialising in a new area with a different client group; or making some bold choices, such as leaving behind one area of our work to pick up something new. I would encourage every SALT to aim high and know that you are so much more capable than you think.

If the field of SSDs inspires you, take up the challenge and keep learning, acquiring new skills, and sharing them with others.

INDEX

AAC 110, 218, 239
ADHD 81, 235
aetiology 6, 9
age of speech sound acquisition *see* developmental norms
anxiety: in child 168, 174, 210; parental 70, 104
articulation disorder: differential diagnosis of 12, 16, 18, 21–6, 33, 213–4; treatment 132–42
ASD 62, 81, 100, 235
ASHA 27, 28, 148

babbling: case history 41; risk factor for SSD 64, 109; therapy 111
backward chaining 128
bilingualism *see* cultural and linguistic considerations
blocks and breaks approach 193–195
body function 10, 68
Bowen, C. 120, 124
BPVS 73, 77

case history taking 39–42
case profile 79–85
CELF–5 73, 74, 76
childhood dysarthria 25, 31, 34
classification of SSD: aetiological 9, 10; level of functioning 10; psycholinguistic 10–12
classroom–based interventions *see* schools

cleft palate: articulation difficulties associated with 163–4; as a specialism 6, 54, 61, 105, 162; feeding, effect on 63; oral examination 57, 60; transcription of speech 53
connected speech: assessment of 45–47; for goal setting 92
consistency of speech: assessment of 42, 43, 46; in CAS 27; in CVI 127–9; in cycles approach 119
consistent phonological disorder 17–18
consonant elicitation 138–141
core vocabulary intervention 126–31
contrastive phonological intervention 114–20
cues: articulation therapy 133, 138; assessment 44, 45, 49, 54; cleft palate therapy 163; CVI 128; DTTC 128; goal–setting 93; minimal pair therapy 115; NDP3 144; PROMPT 150
cultural and linguistic considerations 159–160
cycles approach 119, 150

DDK: assessment of 60, 61; CAS characteristic 29, 31
DEAP 11, 43, 44, 49, 60, 76, 125, 130, 167

developmental dysarthria *see* childhood dysarthria
developmental norms: consonant acquisition 24; phonological processes 15
diagnostic statement 83–5
discharge 180–4
Dodd, B. 10, 11, 13, 14, 17, 33
dosage 175–9
Down's Syndrome 10
DTTC 113, 145–7, 238
dynamic assessment 45, 146
dyslexia 42, 81, 100, 228, 235

early intervention *see* preverbal intervention
Ebbels, S. 205
evidence–based practice 94–5

family history 42, 64, 109
frequency of therapy *see* dosage

games: parent/school lead 105, 212; SALT–lead 116, 158, 178, 186, 197, 199
generalisation: in older children 156, 158; PML 132–6, 141; and rate of progress 177; with TA work 213, 214
goal–setting 91–3
group therapy 191–2
Grunwell, P. 15, 16, 24, 26

hearing status: in case history–taking 39; in therapy prioritisation 188

inconsistent phonological disorder: versus CAS 29–31, 46; characteristics of 19–20; treatment for 125–31; in school–based therapy 214
IEP 92
imitation: in articulation therapy 133; in CAS 29, 36; in case–history taking 41; in CVI 126;
in DTTC 146, 147; in IPD 19
intelligibility: assessment of 41–2, 44, 45–7, 50, 54, 60, 79, 209, 236; in CP 164; in cycles approach 150; EAL 160; enlarged tonsils, effect of 59; and IPD 125, 127; as prioritization criterion 188–9; in report–writing 218; in target–setting 92, 200
intonation: in articulation therapy 135; in ASD 164; assessment of 47, 66; in NDP3 145, 146, 147
integrated phonological awareness (IPA) 149
International Phonetic Alphabet (IPA) 54

knowledge of performance 133, 136

language development: AAC, to enhance 110; at–risk factor for SSD 63, 64; in case history– taking 39; consultative approach, use of 204; therapy to develop 111
Law, J. 98
LEA 217, 221–2, 226; *see also* schools
lexical stress 148
listening skills: assessment of 42; in goal–setting 93; intervention to develop 203; in reports 80, 218
liquids, gliding of 15
literacy 227–31; *see also* schools

McCabe, P. 151
minimal pairs intervention 114–8
metalinguistic approaches 119

motor learning: in DTTC 145; in NDP–3 144; in ReST 147; principles of 134–7; in ultrasound biofeedback 149
movement transitions 145
multidisciplinary working 54, 64; *see also* schools multiple areas of need 161–5
Murray, E. 151

nasality: assessment of 44, 45, 47, 48; in dysarthria 25; transcription of 53, 54, 55, 60, 66 NAPA 76; *see also* phonological awareness
NDP3: description of 143–145, 158; dosage required 176; goal–setting 92; oromotor assessment 60, 61
NIPA 153; *see also* phonological awareness
nurseries 181; *see also* schools; multidisciplinary working

oromotor movements; in CAS 31; and feeding 63; significance of 112–3
oromotor dyspraxia 63
outcome measures 166–8, 210, 240
Ozanne, A. 12

parents 33, 40, 41, 62–6, 69–70, 72; *see also* case history taking; tribunals
PHAB 76
phoneme collapse 13, 17, 50
phonemic transcription *see* transcription; IPA phonetic inventory 117, 118
phonetic placement techniques 138–41
phonetic transcription *see* transcription; IPA

phonological awareness: activities to develop 153–5; assessment of 75–6; IPD 30; literacy development 227–31; schools 203, 211, 214; report–writing 218; *see also* IPA; literacy; NAPA; NIPA; rhyme; syllables
phonological delay: consultative approach 191, 204, 213–214; features of 13–16; overlapping with other SSD subtypes 17–18, 34
PIPA 76
pitch 47, 111, 145, 157, 200
polysyllabic words *see* syllables
pre–verbal interventions 108–13
principles of motor learning *see* motor learning prioritisation 188–190
PROMPT 137, 150
prosody: assessment of 44, 45, 47, 50, 54; CAS, feature of 27, 28, 30, 37; intelligibility, effect on 236
psychosocial aspects 183

ReST 147–9, 176
rate: assessment of 45, 47; CAS, feature of 31; therapy for 200
RCSLT: bilingualism 159; CAS 28, 31, 143, 149; cleft lip and palate 164; hearing loss 6; ROOT 240; SEND support 216, 219; SSD 5, 9, 11, 43, 65, 126, 243; telehealth 196; transcription 54
resonance: in CAS 31; in cleft palate 163; dysarthria 25, 31
report–writing: EHCP 217, 220; tribunals 223–6
rhyme: awareness of 76; principles of working on 209–15

schools: group work 191; therapy in 157–8, 178; tiered approach 203–4; see also EHCP; literacy; tribunals
schwa 54, 84, 148
SENCO 184, 191; see also schools
SEND 216–226
severity rating 50, 79, 80, 81, 83, 188
shaping 138
smoothness 148–149; see also movement transition speech sample: analysis of 49–50; collection of 43–9, 52–6
stimulability 43, 44, 49, 50, 115, 116
Strand, E. 145, 238
suprasegmental features 45, 48, 79, 236; see also pitch; voice; volume
syllables: assessment of awareness 75–6; segmentation of 144; working on 153–4, 199, 112
symptom cluster 62

target selection see goal–setting
teachers see schools
telehealth 196–201
terminology 1, 9, 11, 235–6
tiered approach 203–5, 209–10
timing of therapy 171–4
TPT 43, 44
tribunals 221–6
TROG 73

ultrasound biofeedback therapy 136, 149–50

voice 25, 31, 47, 55, 157
volume 25, 31, 47, 111, 157, 164, 200, 236
vowels: assessment of 44, 48, 49, 56, 66; and CAS 28, 30; and IPD 19, 30; therapy 111, 146, 148

WHO 10
Williams, P. 143

For Product Safety Concerns and Information please contact our EU representative GPSR@taylorandfrancis.com
Taylor & Francis Verlag GmbH, Kaufingerstraße 24, 80331 München, Germany

www.ingramcontent.com/pod-product-compliance
Lightning Source LLC
Chambersburg PA
CBHW060559230426
43670CB00011B/1883